Handbook of Ayurvedic Medicine

Science of Life

The Healing Arts and Sciences - Vol. 3

This series is devoted to books and ensuing media productions dealing with healing methods which accent the self-healing possibilities of the body. The healing methods in these books are based either on serious, developing research, and/or methods which have been tested over centuries and millennia, and, thus, bring again to our awareness healings which were forgotten or covered up by time and "progress". The Publishers are actively looking for manuscripts and for additional members of the Editorial Board, welcoming, among others, physicians and allied health personnel. **Write to:** Grunwald & Radcliff Publishers, a division of Global Communications Associates, Inc., 5049 Admiral Wright Road, #344, Virginia Beach, Va., 23462.

The Handbook of Ayurvedic Medicine
Science of Life

by
Alan K. Tillotson, M.A.
Vaidya Mana Bajra Bajracharya

Grunwald & Radcliff Publishers
Virginia Beach, Va. * Houston, Tex. * Lancaster, Pa. *
Lucerne, Switzerland

Medical Disclaimer

This book describes medical practices used by Ayurvedic doctors practicing under the laws of the government of Nepal. In discussing the use of herbs and medical procedures, there is no intention to diagnose or prescribe, and neither the author nor the Publishers endorse the use of this information for anything except educational purposes. Qualified members of the legally-recognized healing professions who use it professionally, do so at their discretion.

We stress that people who believe they are ill should consult a physician of their choice for diagnosis and treatment.

Library of Congress Cataloging-in-Publication Data

Tillotson, Alan Keith, 1950-
The Handbook of Ayurvedic Medicine *Science of Life*

(The healing arts and sciences, vol. 3)
    Biography: p.
        1. Medicine, Ayurvedic. I. Bajracharya, Mana Bajra. II. Title. III. Series. (DNLM: 1. Medicine, Ayurvedic. WZ 80.5.H6 T578h)
R606. T55   1986   610   86-9927
ISBN 0-915133-09-1
ISBN 0-915133-08-3 (soft)

Printed in the United States of America

Contents

Page

Voices: Robert H, Hall, M.D.; Dr. Michael Tierra. C.A.,   *i*
     N.D.; Janice MacKenzie, LA

Acknowledgements   *iii*

Preface   Jeremy G. Geffen M.D.   *iv*

Forewords   Alan K. Tillotson, Dr. Vasant Lad   *vi*

Introduction   The History of Ayurveda   1

Part One
The Theoretical Basis of Ayurveda

Chapter

One   Fundamental Principles   **13**

Two   Body, Mind and Life   **31**

Part Two
The Practical Basis of Ayurveda

Three   Diagnosis   **53**

Four   Pharmacology and Medicinal Plants   **64**

Five   Diet and Hygiene   **76**

Six   Treatment   **95**

Appendices

One-   Ayurvedic Medicinal Plants   **117**

Two-   Ayurvedic Dietary Prescriptions   **146**

Three-   Ayurveda Resource Directory/Information Exchange   **161**

Four-   Ayurveda Topics on Tape/Advanced Treatment   **167**

Five-   References   **172**

Six-   Bibliography   **174**

Seven-   Index   **178**

Voices From The Experts ...

The Handbook of Ayurvedic Medicine *Science of Life* presents a fine introduction to this system of medicine which is very different from Western medicine. It provides a wealth of information that has previously not been readily accessible to people in the English-speaking countries. Its clarity and readability are a special bonus. The chapter on diet, in conjunction with the appendices, will prove especially valuable to readers interested in applying Ayurvedic principles to their daily lives.

Robert H. Hall M.D.
Wilmington, DE.

It is the first book on Ayurvedic medicine that makes the profound ancient truths of this system practically available and useful to Westerners. I appreciate your finding alternate terms for the difficult to understand Sanskrit language.

Ayurvedic medicine, probably the mother of most Oriental healing disciplines, including Chinese herbology and acupuncture, macrobiotics, etc. ... , is finally available to the professional "holistic" therapist, as well as those who are simply interested in achieving and maintaining health in a common sense, balanced approach to diet and daily living. I think your book is an apt companion to Rudolph Ballentine's book **Diet and Nutrition: A Holistic Approach.**

To the acupuncture therapist and student of traditional Chinese medicine and to the macrobiotic diet advocate, your book should offer a valuable expansion to the Oriental principle of "health as balance".

I find your descriptions of the approach of your teacher, Dr. Mana, as described in your book, in many ways approach my own clinical experience. The approach treats the person as a balance of spiritual-mental and physical qualities and addresses itself to the practical integrative way which should be of practical use for everyone, both professional and lay person.

I have always believed that there is a value to studying with someone who has predigested a difficult concept such as Ayurvedic medicine. The great concepts of Ayurveda are based upon a common sense approach to living and health that has accumulated in the form of a vast storehouse of healing wisdom for over 5,000 years. The descriptions of your studies with the Buddhist Ayurvedic Dr. Mana in Nepal show the tremendous value and potential that Ayurvedic medicine has when and if the Western medical establishment comes around to recognizing it.

Dr. Michael Tierra   C.A., N.D.
Author, The Way of Herbs

This is an excellent, clearly written introduction to Ayurvedic medicine -- I especially love the history of its beginnings and the glimpses of Ayurvedic medical training. Like traditional acupuncture and other natural systems of healing, Ayurveda starts with the macrocosm of the universe and shows how man is just a microcosmic reflection of it. I appreciate that Alan (K.Tillotson) has given us the philosophical and theoretical underpinnings of Ayurveda first, so that we have the appropriate context for the actual medical practices. I thought it was fascinating that both acupuncture and Ayurveda are founded on all-embracing natural laws, just clothed in different language and then divergent in the particulars of diagnosis and treatment. The book is required reading for healers of all persuasions -- particularly those wanting to understanding Eastern forms of medicine.

Janice MacKenzie
Licensed Acupuncturist

ii

Acknowledgements

I wish, first of all, to acknowledge fully the role of my wife Carmelita. To her goes the credit for the needed stimulus to fire my personal growth which has continued unabated since I met her. Her ability to provide conscious direction and psychological support has been nothing short of miraculous.

The faculty of Goddard College, and Bill Meek and Susan Drury in particular, deserve thanks for their professional gui-dance and support when the work was being developed as the basis for my master's thesis.

Dr. Rudolph Ballentine, Drs. Lesley and Michael Tierra, Don Orlik R.Ph., Sumite and the many other teachers and friends at yoga ashrams throughout the world have aided the work in unsuspected ways by simple virtue of their willingness to advise me at critical junctures.

Bronwyn Mills did wonders with preliminary editing, as did Teri Foster in diagramming and layout. Charles Parker did the striking pencil and ink drawing for the cover. Medical illustrator Pat Kenny did the beautiful drawings in the first chapter. All plant drawings in Appendix One were done by Vaidya Mana Bajra Bajracharya.

Alan K. Tillotson, Wilmington

Preface

I first met Vaidya Mana Bajra Bajracharya (or Dr. Mana, as he is more affectionately called by his many patients) while working on a medical expedition to Nepal during the summer of 1984. As an American medical student, I was conducting a research survey of the ancient, traditional forms of medicine which are still being practiced in Nepal.

Dr. Mana's stature and reputation as an Ayurvedic healer are quite reknowned, and it seemed that all of my inquiries about traditional medicine in Nepal sooner or later led directly to his small office near Kathmandu's Mahaboudha Square. So many people knew of Dr. Mana and could relate stories of his impressive ability to cure illnesses when all other treatments had failed. In fact, even the head stewardess on my long Pan Am flight to Nepal -- a German woman who had lived in Nepal for seven years -- enthusiastically told me about the herbal cure for intestinal amoebiasis which she had finally received from Dr. Mana, after she had undergone multiple, unsuccessful treatments with the most powerful modern antibiotics from doctors in both Europe and the United States.

Over the course of four consecutive days I spent numerous hours with Dr. Mana in his clinic. During this time, I was most impressed with Dr. Mana's clear vision and under-standing of the principles and practice of Ayurvedic medicine. He has a wonderful sense of humor, and he is deeply com-mitted to the Buddhist ideals of compassion, loving kindness and relieving human suffering wherever possible. Watching him work with his patients and listening to their stories of how he has helped them, made all of this very evident. Fur-thermore, over time I became convinced that Dr. Mana's profound understanding of human nature -- in addition to his knowledge of anatomy, physiology,

Buddhist philosophy and Ayurvedic medicine -- are gifts which could greatly benefit many others in the world.

It is very important to emphasize that some of Dr. Mana's explanations about particular diseases or their treatments do not make sense within the paradigm of Western medical sci-ence. At times they may even seem to directly contradict ideas which are considered to be basic, or fundamental, scientific facts. The point is, Ayurvedic ideas and principles are often not easily translated directly into Western medical term-inology. And, therefore, the validity or value of these ideas and principles should not be judged, at least initially, by whether or not they appear intuitively or intellectually in accord with our own. Rather, one might consider approaching Ayurveda as a totally new way of understanding not only oneself but the universe as a whole. For Ayurveda is not only a medical science with specific and eminently prac-tical applications, but it is also a philosophy, a way of living, and a "science of life" that has evolved out of direct human experience, insight, and observation of many, many cen-turies. Alan Tillotson's book about Dr. Mana and his unique medical practice is a welcome introduction into the world of Ayurveda and one of its foremost practioners. In addition, the book furthers the possibility that Dr. Mana's vast storehouse of knowledge and understanding may someday become known to all those who could benefit so directly from it. And this, indeed, is a great service.

Jeremy G. Geffen M.D.
La Jolla, CA.

Forewords

In 1976 while traveling across Asia, I suddenly contracted a serious case of dysentery. After three torturous weeks in which Western medicine failed, I took the advice of two experienced travelers and headed to Nepal, where I was given the address of Dr. Mana, a famous herbal doctor in Kathmandu Valley, known for his ability to treat serious intestinal cases such as mine. Dr. Mana, whose full name is Vaidya Mana Bajra Bajracharya, lived up to his reputation by curing my dysentery in a few days. He also administered an herbal tonic which restored my general energy and spirits. I learned that he headed a "Vaidya" or doctor family in Kathmandu. The 46 members of his family live at a large clinic near the king of Nepal's palace. At the clinic, they handled all collecting, preparing and dispensing of herbal medicines according to the ancient medical tradition of Ayurveda. Dr. Mana's older brother was personal physician to the king, as was his father and grandfather. After my treatment, I stayed to study Ayurveda with him at the Mahaboudha clinic.

Dr. Mana said that in the '50s and '60s foreign visitors came to him primarily interested in Buddhism (he is a Vajrayana Buddhist priest). In the early '70s, however, they started asking about treatments and herbal medicines. At first, most people had diarrhea and dysentery, which Ayurveda can easily treat. Gradually, the clinic's reputation increased and a significant percentage of people came for treatment of more serious diseases, especially those which are difficult to cure with Western medicine, such as herpes, breast cancer, asthma, psoriasis, allergies and hepatitis. By 1974 he set aside a small part of the clinic exclusively to treat many patients coming from Germany, France, Italy, the United States, Japan, Russia, etc. During the months I spent at the clinic observing Dr. Mana and his family at work, I had ample opportunity to interview many Westerners who claimed to have been successfully treated.

Near the end of my stay, Dr. Mana asked me to help him edit his manuscript on Ayurvedic dietary practices, which resulted in a small book published in Nepal in 1978.

Shortly after returning to America, I began searching for a school where I could do graduate research in Ayurveda. All schools I investigated limited their approach to anthropology or sociology, except Goddard, a Vermont college based on the philosophy of the great American psychologist John Dewey. It was willing to grant me a master's degree for my research, if I proved to a screening committee that my work would help mankind. The school accepted my idea of returning to Dr. Mana to learn his methods of treating diseases, and I traveled to Kathmandu in the summer of 1980 to resume my studies of Ayurveda. This book is derived largely from my thesis, completed in 1981, along with materials collected in 1983 in Gujarat, India, where I met with Dr. Mana during an Earthwatch expedition.

Ayurveda is making inroads into America, although it has been intensely studied in Germany, Russia, China and Japan for many years. Activity has increased remarkably since 1983, primarily because many long-established yoga ashrams became involved in Ayurvedic medicine. (The ashrams are listed in this book.) It is important to know there are different schools of Ayurveda throughout India, and their understandings and treatment techniques vary. The Nepalese Buddhist tradition of Dr. Mana is a substream in the larger stream of Ayurvedic thought. In southern India, for example, there is a much greater emphasis on cleansing procedures than herbology because of the dry climate and limited vegetation. Nepal, on the other hand, has a vast array of medicinal plants throughout the year in its many climates, and herbology is given a primary importance. Dr. Mana's tradition also requires a deep study of anatomy, rejuvenation therapy, and children's diseases, and is probably unique in that its evolution in these areas has continued from father to son for 700 years. Nepal, fortunately, escaped the political and military battles which raged over India for much of the past 600 years.

The centuries of experience in Dr. Mana's family helped him effectively treat foreigners because many difficulties he encountered were similar to those his family faced when new diseases arose or an important herbal medicine became difficult to obtain. Records of the best ways of meeting new challenges were kept and updated each generation. Still, it took him time to learn to adjust his treatments for quick, effective cures in bodies which were, in his words, "raised under different hygienic circumstances."

Successful treatment also required understanding and cooperation from the new patients, so he had to learn enough Western ideas to explain the Ayurvedic concepts. The difficulties in translating Ayurvedic medical concepts into English are so great that a prominent Ayurvedic scholar from India told a group of Westerners (including myself) it was impossible. Ted Kapchuk, a well-known authority on Chinese medicine, says, "It is impossible to read into the Chinese system the classifications of the West." And "this sort of attempt to impose parallelism on two systems is inappropriate and leads to misunderstanding."

The same caution is needed in Ayurveda, but there are many Ayurvedic terms which can be translated easily because they are close to Western ideas. This is partially true because Ayurveda, far more than Chinese medicine, carefully investigated anatomy and physiology from the time of the ancients. Dr. Mana's use of Western approximations such as "nervous type person" rather than "vata prakruti" enabled him to quickly and effectively deal with patients. I believe any misunderstandings which result are minor compared to the distraction of attempting to grasp Sanskrit terms in an introductory book such as this. So I used his approximations.

In the first five chapters I tried to provide a solid foundation by emphasizing key concepts of this unique and completely natural system of medicine. I hope that in so doing, the idea of "balanced health" -- too often a vague concept -- will have a more precise meaning. The basic ideas are tied together in the last chapter to show how and why Ayurveda, perhaps the oldest medical system on our planet, can treat some of our most serious diseases. The treatments given are based on traditional Ayurvedic knowledge, interpreted in the light of Dr. Mana's more than 40 years of clinical experience. If the economic, political and psychological barriers to the free spread of Ayurveda are removed, and none erected, untold numbers of suffering people can benefit. It is for them that this book is written.

Alan Keith Tillotson, M.A.
Wilmington, DE.
Christmas Day 1985

As an Ayurvedic physician with over 18 years of experience, I feel strongly that Ayurveda encompasses not only a medical science, but a universal religion and philosophy of life.

Ayurveda believes every individual is a creation of the cosmos. An individual is an indivisible, total being. In the pure cosmic consciousness there is Purusha and Prakriti. Prakriti is female energy, which is creativity. She does the divine dance of creation before Purusha, whose role is solely witnessing creation. Prakriti, out of her love, manifests into intelligence, the center of individuality (ego) and three basic attributes (satva, rajas and tamas). From satva she manifests into five sense organs, five motor organs and five basic elements (ether, air, fire, water and earth). In the human body the smaller and larger spaces are ether. Without ether there is no freedom to move and grow. All voluntary and involuntary

ix

movements in the tissues, organs and cells are governed by the air. Fire is responsible for metabolism, digestion, absorption and assimilation. Water governs nutrition, and all solid tissues are the earth element. Out of these five basic elements three biological humors are formed (tri-dosha). These are: Vata (ether & air), Pitta (fire & water) and Kapha (water & earth). These three doshas govern all physio-pathological and psychosomatic changes in the body.

At fertilization, the permutations and combinations of these three doshas determine the individual's constitution (psychosomatic temperament) or "Prakruti". These three doshas are dynamic energies which act and react with the external environment and create internal changes. Diet, lifestyle and changes in season also produce changes in the bodily doshas and may disturb their balance, producing psychosomatic disorders. To correct these disturbances one has to follow proper diet, herbs, cleansing and lifestyle, specific to one's own constitution. Ayurveda provides a complete program for rejuvenation and longevity.

The Handbook of Ayurvedic Medicine *Science of Life* is well-researched and a practical study of Ayurvedic principles. Open-minded study of this material will be of great benefit to the reader.

Dr. Vasant Lad
Director, School of Ayurvedic Medicine
Santa Fe, N.M.

Introduction

The History of Ayurveda

"Anatomy and physiology like some aspects of chemistry were by-products of Hindu medicine. As far back as the sixth century B.C., Hindu physicians described ligaments, sutures, lymphatics, nerve plexus, fascia, adipose and vascular tissue, mucus and synovial membranes ... They understood remarkably well the process of digestion ... (and) the functions of gastric juices ... Sushruta, professor of medicine in the University of Benares, wrote down in Sanskrit a system of diagnosis and therapy ... (which) deals at length with surgery, obstetrics, diet, bathing, drugs, infant feeding and hygiene and medical attention."

Will Durant
Historian

"Ayurveda" is the name given the scientific art of medicine developed by the ancient Indo-Nepalese civilization of the Himalayas. Ayurveda (ayur = life, veda = knowledge) is best translated as "knowledge of life". The earliest reliable records of such knowledge are in the four vedas, or holy books of the Aryans.[1] Within the Vedas, compiled circa 5,000 - 3,000 B.C., is a great deal of medical knowledge in the forms of hymns, liturgical formulas and philosophical treatises. The *Artharva Veda* especially contains many medical references and is, therefore, considered the precursor of Ayurveda.

For the most part, the medical knowledge of those times was a mixture of religious and medical; for example, the

1

Artharva Veda attributes the cause of diseases to the workings of demons, sorcerers and various non-human entities, while encouraging the use of amulets, charms and incantations.[2] In the following millennia, circa 2,500 - 1, 500 B.C., evidence of important medical progress can be seen at the two most important excavation sites in the Indus Valley -- Harappa and Mohenjo-daro. Houses had fresh water tanks, bathrooms and drains. Sanitation was important and simple herbal compounds were used, testifying to the existence of more than superficial medical knowledge.[3] However, it seems clear this early knowledge was not codified into an easily intelligible or scientific form. Instead, it was handed down from person to person and generation to generation as part of the religious and philosophical teachings at ashrams of Brahman scholars and priests, or homes of other Hindu castes.

The Origin of Ayurveda

When the *Upanishads* (the more philosophical writings following the *Vedas*) were compiled, an age of high intellectual and spiritual development flourished in Indo-Nepal, and an ordered presentation of medicine naturally arose. Our knowledge of the events then (circa 700 B.C.) comes primarily from the *Charaka Samhita,* the medical encyclopedia of the physician Charaka, who lived c. 123 A.D.[4] Charaka describes in detail the formal origin of Ayurveda at a major spiritual and medical conference in the Himalayan mountains circa 700 B.C. A large part of Charaka's encyclopedia, in fact, was written by a student physician, named Agnivesa, during that conference.

The philosophical and spiritual values of the sages and medical scholars at this conference were debated until certain principles were adopted as the theoretical foundation of Ayurveda. The most important principles were Vata, Pitta, and Kapha, a triadic division of the physical and metaphysical universe derived from the traditional Hindu cosmology. These three great principles became the mental framework for under-

2

standing how the human body works. The ancient sage-scholars considered these principles absolute, much as we consider space and time to be absolute truths.

These refer to the idea that all physical reality is an interplay between creation (Kapha), destruction (Pitta), and order or intelligence (Vata). To this day, an understanding of these inde-pendent principles is the basis of Ayurveda.

The Eight Principles of Ayurveda

After the Great Conference, areas of medical knowledge were split into eight main divisions, called the "Ashtanga (eight-armed) Ayurveda". They are:

1. Internal Medicine
2. Surgery
3. Eyes, Ears, Nose, Mouth and Throat
4. Children's Diseases
5. Toxicology
6. Rejuvenation Therapy
7. Semen and Uterus Purification
8. Spiritual Healing

Internal Medicine

Kayachikitsa Tantra is the science of general treatment or internal medicine. The Vaidya (Ayurvedic doctor) presiding over internal medicine at the Great Conference was Punarvasu Atreya. The treatise compiled by his student Agnivesa, the *Agnivesa Samhita,* is the most reliable record of Atreya's life and work. It is exceptionally valuable because it is composed of extensive dialogues between Atreya, who taught orally, and his disciples. This work was incorporated by Charaka in the *Charaka Samhita* and the original does not exist. A copy of the *Harita Samhita,* by another of Atreya's students, was published in Sanskrit about 50 years ago, but there are doubts about its authenticity, though it's the first description of some important medical approaches still used. [5] A copy of the *Bhela*

Samhita, written by yet a third student of Atreya, was recently retrieved in extremely poor condition in southern India.

The school of Punarvasu Atreya continued to produce many important Vaidyas after his death. The most important are: Dridhabala in the 2nd century A.D.; Vagbhata in the 5th century A.D.; Chakrapani in the 10th century A.D.; Vijayaraksita in the 13th century A.D.; Sarngadhara in the 14th century A.D., and Bavamisra in the 16th century A.D.

Dridhabala is known for reviving *Charaka Samhita* and adding chapters. Vagbhata taught Ayurveda in Tibet, where much of the medical science is based on his teachings. He wrote two books detailing the fundamentals of the eight divisions. Chakrapani wrote a valuable text on using refined minerals in Ayurvedic medicines. Vijayaraksita wrote the *Madhava Nidama*, a basic text on diagnosis, and Sarngadhara's text, the *Sarngadhara Samhita,* describes specific medicines for specific diseases, while Bavamisra contributed to Ayurvedic botany. This brief list shows the school of Punarvasu Atreya consistently developed internal medicine. It is the only division of Ayurvedic medicine which maintained a tradition of practical training.

Surgery
Salya Tantra is defined as "surgery". Dhanvantari Divodasa was the original presiding Vaidya over this division and many of his disciples wrote important works on the subject. The disciple Susruta wrote the best and most reliable research work on surgery with commentaries on the other divisions. Its intelligence and comprehensiveness rivals the *Charaka Samhita* in value to Ayurveda students. It is clear from the *Susruta Samhita* that ancient surgeons skillfully used delicate surgical instruments and performed many difficult operations such as abdominal surgery, chest surgery, cranial sections, removal of bladder stones and plastic surgery of the nose.

The ingenuity of the ancient surgical techniques is astounding: patients were given animal blood to drink in cases of excessive bleeding [6] ; ants were put on the perforated body areas and allowed to bite firmly, then separated at the head, leaving unique stitches, and elaborate pre- and postoperative care was given. [7]

Jivaka was a famous surgeon from Dhanvantari's school, living during the time of Buddha. Jivaka's association with Buddha prompted much information to be written about him in the Tibetan and Nepalese Buddhist literature. For instance, he is said to have invented an x-ray-like jewel derived from a now unknown form of wood, successfully used for internal diag-noses. He was famed for his work in brain surgery, in addition to other areas of Ayurveda.

The techniques developed in the ancient surgery school are not practiced, although in Nepal a vestigial form survives within the Nau caste of barbers. Some Naus perform minor oper-ations, but they are often ill-qualified, with no serious training.

Eyes, Ears, Nose, Mouth and Throat

Janaka was the original presiding Vaidya over the eyes, ears, nose, mouth and throat division. He also was known as Videha, and composed important books under this name, the lost *Videha Tantra* being the most important. However, the *Susruta Samhita* thoroughly covers Janaka's work and, so, is considered the most reliable source work for the division.

Children's Diseases

Kasyapa was the original presiding Vaidya over the children's diseases division. A close student wrote the only valid text of this division, the *Kasyapa Samhita,* dealing with disease treatments for children, mothers and wet nurses. The practical training in this division is carried on primarily in the Buddhist priest class.

5

Toxicology

Kasyapa Rishi headed the toxicology division. His original text, the *Kasyapa Samhita* (not to be confused with the book of the same title in the children's diseases division) is lost. References to the text are in the pertinent chapters of the *Susruta Samhita* and the *Ashtanga Hridaya*.

Rejuvenation

Rejuvenation and health maintenance had no presiding head or primary reference text. In general, the material from this division is a major subject in the texts of internal medicine. Through the centuries, the rishis (learned sages) made tremendous progress, and the principles of preparing mineral medicines are based on their research. In the 1st century A.D., this division was divided into Hindu and Buddhist schools, headed by Adityanath and Nagarjuna, respectively. Almost all of their work, and the work of their highly respected lineages, are still available, and constitute one of the great untapped cultural heritages of Indo-Nepal.

Rejuvenation therapy is usually practiced on older people. The body is cleansed with enemas, purgatives, emetics, steam baths and so forth. Adjunct procedures include mental disciplines and meditation for calming the mind. Then patients are given dosages of potent Ayurvedic rejuvenation medicines. These medicines restore elasticity to the body and replace important nutrients and minerals depleted with age. The dosage, diet, method of administration and timing depend on the patient's condition and the potency of the medicine used.

Uterus and Semen Purification

The science of uterus and semen purification did not have a separate existence, but developed with close ties to the schools of internal medicine and rejuvenation. It tried to avoid unhealthy births through medicines which purified semen and the uterus before conception.

6

Spiritual Healing

Scientific and religious elements of Ayurveda were not separate before the Great Conference. Afterward, most religious, spiritual and psychological elements were put in the spiritual healing division, generally given less importance by the general medical practitioners, and considered the domain of priests and holy men (also called Vaidyas). Its treatments are reserved usually for cases where the principles of Vata, Pitta and Kapha cannot be seen operating after diagnosis.

One such spiritual therapy is mantra, or sound therapy. Audible and inaudible sounds are believed to alter the flow of pranic (life) energy through vibrations produced by a trained person chanting a mantra, affecting sense organs and the nervous system. Vowels are considered to be a female sound and consonants to be male because vowels require a relaxation of the body to sound, while consonants require a tension. In ancient times the religious practitioners spent lifetimes determining the effects sounds produced in the physical body. They recorded many mantras still used today. This is an extremely difficult art to master, but there are numerous records of mantra practitioners who cured paralysis and other nervous disorders with powerful vocal vibrations.

Another spiritual healing procedure is bali or offering. This treatment prescribes different foods and medicines for diseases as in standard treatment. In bali the foods and medicines are first offered to the patient. He is told to touch them with his hands and then dispose of them in a garden, crossroads or cemetery. This treatment attracts a negative vibration or unknown subtle disease agent from the body. It is generally used in mental rather than purely physical diseases.

Ayurvedic spiritual healers claim knowledgeable applications of spiritual healing therapies sometimes have had an almost miraculous effect in cases of paralysis, children's diseases and mental cases where traditional therapies have failed.

7

Medical Instruction

In ancient times, it was possible to study Ayurveda in an ashram or at the home of a Vaidya family. An ashram is a building dedicated to religious practice and secular education. Ayurvedic ashrams were usually in tranquil locations near rivers or forests. Medical instruction in the ashrams was reserved for students from the highest castes, the Brahmans (the Hindu priest class) or Ksetriyas (the caste of the ruler's family). Education in the homes of private Vaidyas was for members of tribes who, living in their small indigenous villages or settlements, could not provide for an ashram. For this reason, the education of an ashram was usually superior to the one from a private home. The Indian and Nepalese governments still recognize both forms of education.

People selected by the guru (teacher) of an ashram to become medical students were initiated in a religious ceremony known as "Upanayama Samskara". The students were 10 to 12 years old when they entered the ashram and could expect to spend 12 to 18 years under a single teacher before completing their studies. In general, students had to study 12 years to become a Vaidya, and six more years to specialize in one of the eight Ayurvedic divisions.

Life in a Medical Ashram

Life in a medical ashram is disciplined and its pattern today is much the same as in ancient times. Students must get up at dawn each day, move their bowels, bathe, pray and meditate. They then spend three hours with their teacher memorizing lessons. This is followed by a very simple lunch in which meat, garlic, onions and intoxicating beverages are strictly prohibited because they detract from the meditative atmosphere considered necessary for deep study. Following the meal the students can rest briefly. They return to class at noon and continue studying for a minimum of three hours. After this, they are free until dinner which is always served before sunset. Memorization and book reading are prohibited after

8

dinner and students are encouraged, instead, to discuss and debate the subjects. Debate was considered a high art by the writers of the ancient medical classics. And the medical art was developed, in large part, through scholars' debates and discussions. This skill also was needed to help establish a good community reputation. Finally, on the first and eighth days of the lunar calendar -- holy days in the Hindu religion -- students collect plants and herbs and help prepare medicines.

Subjects and Methods of Study

Instruction in Ayurveda, regardless of the branch, requires a scientific form. The methodology is based on: 1) direct observation; 2) applying deductive, inductive and analogical reasoning to analyze, and 3) paying attention to the known authoritative knowledge (textbooks) on the subject. Alternately, the student must: 1) start with the textbook knowledge, 2) follow this study with direct observation, and 3) submit the facts to analysis using deductive, inductive and analogical reasoning. Conclusions are then subject to experiments.

Also, all medical students are educated in Hindu literature, philosophy and religion. Perhaps, the most important subject is Sanskrit. Because all the Sanskrit texts are medical texts, students automatically enhance their understanding of anatomy, physiology, botany, pharmacology, hygiene and diet during their language study. Finally, students must help care for patients.

Practical anatomy and physiology study began by soaking corpses in water for seven days under the shade of a tree in a forest, and watching the body's layers peel methodically. This is still considered a practical method because the students see body separations as naturally differentiated. In skin study, for instance, this method allows the clear differentiation of seven layers. Nerves and blood vessels also stand out clearly.[8]

9

The botany and pharmacology studies also are conducted where students can collect plants and herbs. The study of diet and hygiene is incorporated in students' daily lives.

After six years of education in Sanskrit and general medicine, students can join advanced medical classes. Here they are instructed in the eight branches of Ayurveda. Advanced study requires about six years, and during this time students must memorize and recite by heart many of the most difficult and important stanzas in the textbooks. After 12 years of study, the students receive the title of "Vaidya" and government permission to practice medicine.

Postgraduate Study

If a student specializes in one of the eight Ayurvedic divisions, he must study for six more years, usually at another ashram. In ancient times, each division was taught by different ashram schools, with each having a founding head and primary text. Schools also had vast selections of specialized texts written by their Vaidyas throughout the centuries.

The amazing achievements of these ancient schools are a matter of historical record. Medical students came from all parts of the Eastern world for advanced study in the most famous ashram schools, such as the ones in Takashila and Benares. Ayurvedic Vaidyas taught in Greece, China, Tibet, Persia and Arabia. The traditional medicine of these countries still owes a debt to Ayurveda.[9]

Home Study

Each Indian and Nepalese tribe has its own culture, language and close-knit community. Within each community are families of Vaidyas, trained generation-by-generation through the family. In ancient times, this study was well-organized, just as in the ashrams. Children chosen between ages 8 and 12 were initiated through a religious ceremony known as "vratabandha" or "chudakarma". Working with their Vaidya fathers and grandfathers, they were educated first in their native language and then in Sanskrit. They watched the round-the-clock treatment given in the family clinic: diagnosis, treatment, preparation of medicines, etc., receiving clinical experience along with their studies in anatomy, physiology, botany, pharmacology, hygiene, diet, etc. At ages 20 to 25 they became assistants, handling patients alone and only requiring advice from their elders in complicated cases.

Postgraduate study also was possible because many families specialized in one or two of the eight Ayurveda branches. They might, for example, have their own meditation system to develop spiritual healing abilities, or advanced training in herbology. Sometimes, family members were sent to ashrams for postgraduate study.

Historical Development
Because of the intensive work done at and after the Great Conference, the ashram schools enjoyed tremendous development before the birth of Christ. From the 1st century through the Medieval time, the siddhas (saints) introduced many powerful medicines to find the physical means to delay or overcome death, and they revolutionized medicine. The success of their potent medicines gradually eroded surgical discipline. People became afraid of major operations and the practice of surgery declined markedly.

The Medieval Time (First - Tenth Centuries)
India's medieval time was one of great social crisis, with continual wars and long struggles for political power. Inevitably, the work of the great siddhas, or saint-physicians, declined; their valuable work was preserved only in books, and the tradition of practical training was broken. The reputation and achievements of Ayurveda were weakened and corrupted in the hands of physicians who practiced without adequate study or clinical preparation.

Moslem invasions beginning in the 11th century A.D. were responsible for the destruction of valuable medical texts.

Traditional practices and important developments were discouraged by invaders, and ensuing British rule did not improve the situation. Today, there are many Ayurvedic ashrams in India and Nepal, but with few exceptions, the education is no longer as it was in ancient times.

Modern Developments

Home training in Ayurveda continues. Among the Newars -- one of the first civilized tribes in the Kathmandu Valley -- there are, for example, several Vaidya families who are successful and respected. Buddhist Newars, required to stay under the discipline of monasteries, are especially well known for their high education standards. They follow the methods and texts of the ancient schools. Their centuries of unbroken medical work created successful and unique treatments.

On the other hand, the Vaidya families in other tribes have let their advance work decline. There has always been a great temptation to get involved in simple symptomatic treatment and many children from the traditional families have assumed the title "Vaidya" without the proper training. This abuse, stemming back to past centuries, badly hurt the reputation of Ayurveda home study.

Politics and the decline of the ashram and home study schools brought Ayurvedic knowledge to a standstill until the late 19th century. Fortunately, much advanced work survived in private libraries of families and religious orders; and, since the end of World War I, the Vaidyas have focused on reconstruction and development in India and Nepal. The Indian government appointed special committees to examine the problems of Ayurveda. New schools, including Ayurvedic hospitals, and the increased opportunities for communication and interchange of knowledge among world medical communities, are gradually favoring the advancement of Ayurvedic medicine.

Part One
The Theoretical Basis of Ayurveda

Chapter One
Fundamental Principles

"The real key to health is to learn how to maintain the integrity of the interactions of three major networks -- the central nervous system, the endocrinological, and the immunological network."

Dr. Robert Good, M.D.
Former Director, Sloan-Kettering Institute, N.Y.

The 6th century B.C. was a time of man's intellectual awakening worldwide. In the East, Gautama Siddharta founded Buddhism and Mahavira Jnatiputra founded Jainism. The Chinese classics, the *Tao Te Ching* by Lao-tse and the *Confucian Five Classics* and *Four Books,* were being written, as were the Persian scriptures.[10] The science of yoga developed centuries earlier in India, and was well systemized and widely taught by this time. The Hebrew fathers were working on the Torah in Babylon, Pythagoras was teaching mathematics and philosophy, and Greek physicists along the Lydian coast were doing scientific or practical work. The occult philosopher Mark Edmund Jones says all these events "give the modern student every reason to suspect that there were intellectual no less than trade contacts in all directions."[11] Ayurveda was born in this world context.

The Purpose and Methodology of Ayurveda

The all important medical encyclopedia, the *Charaka Samhita,* provides the philosophy and principles of Ayurveda through a series of dialogues recorded at the Great Medical Conference of 700 B.C. And here each new student of Ayurveda must rediscover the purpose and meaning of this ancient medical science. We can more fully appreciate the humanitarian purpose of Ayurveda knowing the original account of the first meeting of the Ayurveda founders:

Virtuous sages, having compassion on ill people, gathered at the side of the Himalayas for a medical conference.
Charaka Samhita Sutra Asthana 1:7

The virtuous sages discussed health, which is so very important for religious practice, business, happiness in life and emancipation. They realized that the many diseases which confronted humans were a serious problem, causing the destruction of their lives and welfare. So, they asked, what was the solution for controlling diseases and creating health? Thus, in a peaceful mood, they began to meditate on a solution.
Charaka Samhita Sutra Asthana 1:16

The sages, through their contemplation, found the solution through an understanding of problems of reality based on:
1. The assimilating tendencies of similar objects (Samanya)
2. The separating tendencies of dissimilar objects (Vishesha)
3. The nature of physical properties (Guna)
4. The nature of substance (Dravya)
5. The actions of objects according to their properties (Karman)
6. The laws controlling the relationships of objects to their properties (Samavaya)
Charaka Samhita Sutra Asthana 1:28

14

The philosophical terms in the last quote are tools the sages used in exploring diseases and the body's functioning. For example, samanya and vishesha (1 and 2 above) were the basis for understanding how foods and medicines with given qualities (3 above) would affect the body. The ancient methodology was realistic and experiential and would satisfy many criteria of modern science. But the underlying definitions of health and disease vary completely with modern concepts.

Before going into this in detail, keep in mind R. Buckminster Fuller's words:

"While it takes but meager search to discover that many well known concepts are false, it takes considerable search and even more careful examination of one's own personal experience and inadvertently spontaneously reflexing to discover that there are many popular and even professionally unknown, yet, nonetheless fundamental, concepts to hold true in all cases and that have already been discovered by as yet obscure individuals. That is to say, that many scientific generalizations have been discovered but have not yet come to the attention of what we call the educated world at large, thereafter to be incorporated tardily within the formal education process, and even more tardily within the formal political-economic affairs of everyday life. Knowledge of the existence and comprehensive significance of these as yet popularly unrecognized laws is the requisite to the solution of many of the unsolved problems now confronting society. Lack of knowledge of the solution often leaves humanity confounded when it need not be." [12]

A Modern Look at an Ancient System

There are many barriers to a practical understanding of an ancient system of thought. Perhaps the greatest barrier is that it developed in a culture removed from us by thousands of years and the distance of half a world. Our ideas provide the framework of our understanding. For example, we may think we are talking about the same thing when we translate Sanskrit words such as "life" or "body," but we might have totally disparate notions. And our assumptions are generally so deeply entrenched in our consciousness as to make them invisible.

To approach Ayurveda intelligently, then, we must have some idea of both our own assumptions about the nature of body and life, and those of Ayurveda. Furthermore, we must be willing to relinquish, at least temporarily, our preconceptions while learning about Ayurveda -- much as a mathematician must let go of his thoroughly ingrained ideas about straight lines and planes when studying non-Euclidian geometry. To do otherwise will lead to a confused or partial understanding.[13] In addition a spiritual component -- a compassion beyond ordinary thought -- is necessary to the deep affinity for and internalization of Ayurveda's basic purpose and principles, which leads to practical results in one's daily life.

Students might find another approach through the principle of faith of virtually all Ayurvedic doctors in India and Nepal, that ancient founders of Ayurveda were sages who could consciously control many of their internal body functions. Students with sufficient experience in any of the widespread meditation systems can recreate the inner experiences which led to the development of the Ayurvedic principles of body and mind. This is because, at the intermediate and advanced stages of meditation, one experiences the body as a matrix of interrelated energies. For this reason, many teaching parables of Ayurveda stress the inward journey as indispensable to complete understanding of Ayurveda. But we should not think of Ayurveda as a mystical science because it is a very practical system for balancing and healing the body.

16

We are fortunate in studying Ayurveda that the ancient practitioners left voluminous records of the concepts and principles. Life was defined most often as the combination of body, organized perceptions and mind.[14] Each of these terms was further defined and expanded through practical usefulness. For instance, "mind" was defined according to its attributes (purity, aggressiveness and lethargy), and its faculties (such as understanding and memory). The body, on the other hand, was considered a materialization controlled by the three universal metaphysical principles / Vata (order, intelligence), Pitta (destruction) and Kapha (creation), the cornerstones of Ayurvedic thought. The texts, notably the *Charaka Samhita,* outline the unceasing questioning about obtaining happiness, health and longevity that enhanced Ayurveda's understanding and practical application.

Alan K. Tillotson, M.A., spent several years studying with Vaidya Mana Bajra Bajracharya, director of the Ayurveda section of the Royal Nepalese Academy of Science and Technology. Dr. Mana and his family operate an Ayurvedic clinic with the legal support of the Nepalese government. The healer has an internationally-respected reputation for healing people who were unsuccessfully treated by Western doctors. Below, and in other sections of the book, Tillotson uses Dr. Mana's own words to describe Ayurveda diagnoses and treatments.

DR. MANA: "I don't know why, but in 1973 or 1974 people began to become interested in traditional medicine. At first, it was only a few people seeking treatment, asking if I had medicine. After I would prescribe for them and they were cured, they would tell their friends. Now I have Western patients every day. When I saw how many people were interested in herbal treatments, I decided to concentrate on teaching these people.

17

"I stopped most of my other teaching activities and opened a section of our clinic for Westerners. The travelers come here mostly with parasite problems, which Ayurveda can easily cure. In this way, people were impressed. They began to discover that Ayurveda can cure diseases for which they have no effective medicine in the West -- asthma, hepatitis, arthritis, multiple sclerosis, herpes. I was surprised when these patients said they had no success in their treatment in Europe for these diseases.

"In the beginning, I had to concentrate on understanding the Western body types and psychology. To treat properly, I have to be able to determine the patient's body type. If I fail, my medicine will not work. Having developed under different hygienic conditions, the Western body is completely different from the Nepalese. At first, I had to be slow and careful in my treatment, especially in figuring their immunity capacity and ability to handle my medicines."

The Three Fundamental Principles

To fully grasp the great trichotomy of Vata, Pitta and Kapha, it is necessary to realize these terms cut through ordinary conceptions and categories of thought.[15] Like the Hindu Five Element Theory from which they are derived, and like modern space and time, they are at once profoundly simple and profoundly difficult.

We can see that life and health depend on ordinary processes such as inhalation and exhalation of air, intake and digestion of food, and waste excretion. When we try to understand how to inhale and exhale, how and what to eat, and what occurs during digestion, we see many intricate principles. Ancient Ayurvedic doctors recognized the need for

18

common principles to order their thinking, and believed these principles should proceed from their intuitive understanding of the universal to the specific and practical. So they created their triune principles of Vata, Pitta and Kapha.

These three terms have different meanings at different levels of reality. As abstract principles they have one meaning, as material processes another, and as physiological processes still another. It is very important, therefore, to keep these understandings distinct.

At the highest level, the body is seen as a materialization caused by the interplay of three fundamental forces: creation (Kapha); destruction (Pitta) and order or intelligence (Vata). Susruta says: "Vata, Pitta and Kapha are the cause of the body. They are everywhere in the body. In the balanced state they keep the body."

Susruta Samhita Sutra Asthana 21:3

At the next or universal level, these abstractions have concrete correspondences with physical phenomena, and here Ayurveda assumes microcosm and macrocosm. We are the universe and the universe is us. Destruction (Pitta) is represented in the skies by the sun, whose light and heat energize all things on our planet. Similarly, creation (Kapha) is represented by the moon, whose cyclical pull on the earth's fluid system - its oceans - regulates the supply of life-giving water to its people. Order and intelligence (Vata) is rep-resented by the wind (breath, prana, spirit), whose subtle influence is the controlling essence of life:

As the moon, the sun and the air maintain Earth by their energies of creation, destruction and diffusion (of heat and moisture), so do Kapha, Pitta and Vata maintain life.

Susruta Samhita Sutra Asthana 21:6

19

KAPHA, or Creation

"KAPHA" is Sanskrit for "creation". This is the universe as manifestation or matter. Applied to medicine, this principle controls nutrient supply for birth, growth and cell repair. Kapha refers to absorption, as demonstrated universally by the moon's pull on the Earth's oceans. Kapha discords are a large class, all relating to an excess of assimilation, growth, sluggishness, excess mucus exudation and blocked lymphatic ducts. When the body's Kapha or nutritive energy is balanced there is always a good supply of nutrients in the arteries for distribution to the cells. Charaka says:

Kapha has the properties of being heavy, cold, soft, oily, sweet viscous and stable.
Charaka Samhita Sutra Asthana 1:60.

Kapha in the balanced state supplies the body's nutritive energy, and in the overbalanced state causes diseases. The nutritive energy of Kapha is called "oja" in the body, and its overbalanced form is called "salty mucus".
Charaka Samhita Sutra Asthana 17:116.

Kapha or nutritive energy disorders involve overactivity or dysfunction in the large mucus membrane lining the alimentary canal (FIGURE 1), and an improper amount or quality of nutrients in the arteries. In Ayurveda this overactivity indicates simultaneous overbalance in cellular absorption. Because Kapha or nutritive energy overbalance invariably produces waste mucus, this symptom is a primary indicator of Kapha or nutritive energy disorders.

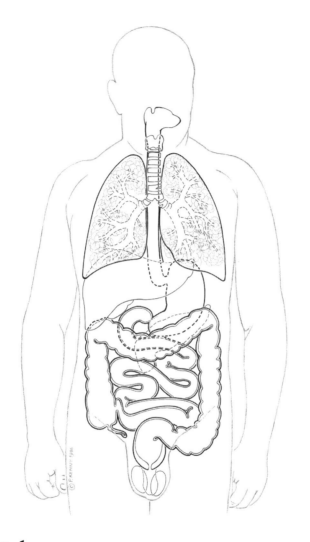

Figure 1.
The principle of creation, KAPHA, is represented
in the physical body by the nutritive energy, which
assimilates and prepares nutrients for supply to
every part of the body.

PITTA, or Destruction

"PITTA" is the Sanskrit term for the principle of "destruction", seeing the universe as energy heat, light, radiation, etc. And in medicine it is metabolic energy. Just as creation and destruction are complimentary processes, so are metabolism and absorption. To demonstrate this, Ayurvedic teachers have students boil food in water to see how fire (a form of Pitta) dissolves the food until it attaches itself to water (a form of Kapha). A similar process occurs inside the alimentary canal, but the "fires" are the digestive ferments of colorful hue, yellow bile being the most obvious. These are well known in the West, of course, but Ayurveda often applies this knowledge differently to health.

In practice, Pitta or metabolic disorders involve overactivity in the blood circulation, which controls heat distribution through dilating and constricting the capillaries (FIGURE 2):

Pitta has the properties of being hot, oily, powerful, liquid, sour, quick moving, and pungent.
Charaka Samhita Sutra Asthana 1:60.

Pitta controls body heat causing metabolism and digestion. When Pitta is overbalanced, it causes diseases.
Charaka Samhita Sutra Asthana 17:115.

Pitta or metabolic disorders are a large class, all relating to digestion and metabolism. Just as an improperly burning candle flame produces smoke, improper body metabolism creates toxic waste. These wastes are usually acids which must be excreted from the body. These toxins are called Pitta "doshas" (metabolic energy defects) in Ayurveda. And if the body can't get rid of them, they accumulate (especially in the veins) and cause the characteristic symptoms of Pitta overbalance: inflammation, hot flashes, infections and rapid tissue decay.

22

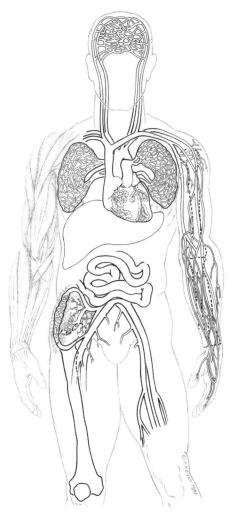

Figure 2.
The principle of destruction, PITTA, is represented in the physical body by the metabolic energy, which generates heat and energy for the
body.

VATA, or Order

"VATA" is Sanskrit for "order". It is the universe seen as the movement of creation and destruction as they continually transform each other. Vata keeps the other two processes from becoming chaotic. In Ayurveda these three principles are seen as truths of all material and mental phenomena.[16]

Vata or nervous energy regulates respiration, perception, voluntary and involuntary movement, and movement of body products such as blood, lymph, nerve impulses, etc. It is the activating and ordering agent of life:

Vata has the properties of being dry (rough), cold, light, fine, movable, non-viscous and harsh.
Charaka Samhita Sutra Asthana 1:59.

Vata causes all body activities and functions. These functions are "pranas" (life currents). Overbalanced Vata causes diseases and balanced Vata results in health.
Charaka Samhita Sutra Asthana 17:117.

Vata is more difficult to understand than Pitta or Kapha because it is linked closely with *prana*, the life current or life force. Ancient sages have described Vata as a god of the universe, external wind which blows down trees, profound currents of prana which sustain and regulate the body, and energy which can cause disease in the body and regulate sensory perception and movement. Vata is hard to understand through scientific or empirical means.

Ayurveda's founders derived their concepts of Vata from meditation. Usually, after years of yoga or meditation, a student becomes aware of an internal energy resembling light, heat, color, etc., linked to breath. With inhalation and exhalation, this energy circulates through the body, flowing along channels and penetrating every cell. The prana controls the nerves (FIGURE 3), especially the autonomic nervous system, and all movement in the body and consciousness.

24

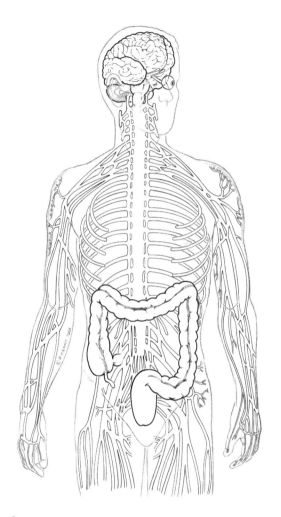

Figure 3.
The universal principle of order, VATA, is
represented in the physical body by the nervous
energy, which directs all the body's movement and
metabolic activities. It connects the brain to the
mind through prana.

25

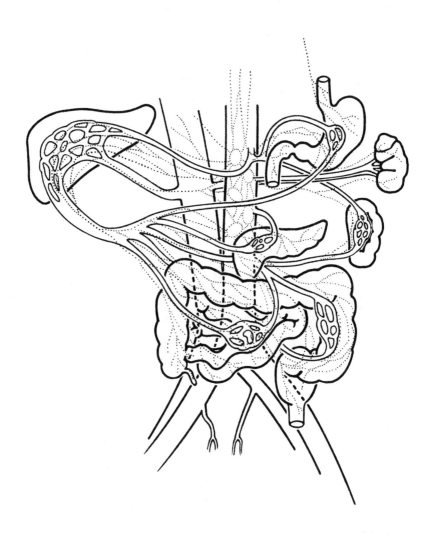

Figure 4.
At the level of individual organs, VATA is the
nerve or prana supply, KAPHA is the nutrients
brought in by the arteries, and PITTA is the
venous and lymphatic drainage of metabolic by-
products.

A proper flow of prana is necessary to make any body part active. Finally, the prana can lead the thinking consciousness to deeper levels of the mind.

For these reasons, Ayurveda maintains it is impossible to separate wind or breath from the nervous system. On a mundane level, the nervous system requires oxygen to survive, and any irregularity in our thinking, perception or voluntary movements involves irregularities in breathing. Nervous energy and prana are manifestations of Vata at different levels of understanding.

Vata or nervous energy disorders are a large class, all characterized by nervous dysfunction, dryness, weakness, putrefactive gases, and irregular mental or organic functions.

Sanskrit	Universal Principle	Energy	Body System	By-Products Of Imbalance
KAPHA	Creation	Nutritive	Nutritive	Mucus
PITTA	Destruction	Metabolic	Blood Circulation	Acids
VATA	Order	Nervous	Nervous	Gases

Figure 5. The correspondences between the three principles and the body.

Energy Inter-Relationships and the Definition of Health

According to Ayurveda, the body's three controlling energy processes, nutritive, metabolic and nervous, are inter-related and interdependent. There are general principles about these processes in medical diagnoses. Nervous energies and nutritive energies balance each other. This means if the nervous energy becomes overbalanced, nutritive energy will decrease and membranes and tissues in the affected area will become dry and undernourished. Similarly, if nutritive energy increases and becomes overbalanced, nervous energy

27

will decrease, and the affected tissue will become heavy and slow, etc. This can be represented as:

Nervous energy <-> Nutritive energy - VATA <-> KAPHA.

If nervous and nutritive energies simultaneously become overactive, metabolic energy will become underactive, causing weakness, cold, etc. This is because the first two, working as a team, control the metabolic energy. In the same way, if metabolic energy becomes overactive, nervous energy and nutritive energy will decrease. This can be represented as:

VATA <-> KAPHA   or   Nervous <-> Nutritive

↓   ↓

PITTA   Metabolic Energies

This is an oversimplification, of course, because there are qualitative and quantitative differences. What is important, however, is the three major energies and their corresponding body processes hold each in homeostasis. When one changes, the others change also.

Health, according to Ayurveda, is a dynamic and intricate state of balance between nutritive, nervous and metabolic energies. Momentary imbalances occur frequently throughout daily life, for example, when we become fearful and our membranes become dry (nervous overbalance) or when we become angry and overheated, losing control of rational processes (metabolic overbalance). In such cases, the body naturally restores balance. A disruption of one or more of the major energies which is so severe the other energies cannot restore homeostasis is, according to Ayurveda, the definition of and primary cause of all diseases.

A big advantage of Ayurveda is it does not depend on sophisticated technical knowledge. It can be integrated with ordinary facts of experience. Ayurveda lists general symptoms of overbalance in the major energies, and if these are bolic and nutritive energy overbalances. Ayurveda stresses that nothing can go wrong in the physical body which cannot be traced by watching these relationships shift.

When nervous energy (Vata) becomes overbalanced, the symptoms are nervousness, lack of clear thoughts, pain, spasm, gas, uncoordinated or shaky movements of limbs, head, eyes, etc. and irregular functioning of muscles, organs, secretions, etc.

When metabolic energy (Pitta) becomes overbalanced, the symptoms are inflammation, hot sensations, fever, infection and rapid tissue decay.

When nutritive energy (Kapha) is overbalanced, the symptoms are abnormal growth, overexudation of mucus and fluids, and overall sluggishness.

If two energies become overbalanced, the person will exhibit both sets of symptoms simultaneously.

Most Ayurvedic treatments attempt to restore homeostasis among the three major energies. Because each major energy is in dynamic relationship with the others, the Ayurvedic Vaidya will strengthen the underbalanced energy (or energies) until it can correct the overbalanced ones. This is the basis of Ayurvedic treatment and will be covered in following chapters.

Summary

According to Ayurvedic teachings, the universe and the body can be understood in terms of three principles: Kapha, Pitta and Vata. Kapha is creation. In the physical body it is nutritive energy, embodied in the nutritive system. Pitta is destruction. In the body this is metabolic energy, embodied in the blood circulatory system. Vata is order. In the body this is nervous energy, embodied in the nervous system. Vata energy is the most subtle of the three, and is known at its higher levels as pranic currents of life energy connecting body with mind.

In the body these three energies hold each other in equilibrium. Health is this moment-to-moment equilibrium. Disease occurs when the body can't naturally restore its balance.

Chapter Two

Body, Mind, and Life

"For three decades Dr. Caroline B. Thomas -- an internist and cardiologist -- had been tracking the physical and mental health of 1,337 Johns Hopkins medical students ... Every year since graduation, Thomas and her colleagues found connections between particular personality traits and specific disorders ... When the study had begun, psychiatrist Dr. Barbara Betz ... divided them into three major temperamental categories. The first group, the 'alphas,' were cautious, steady, self-reliant, slow to adapt and non-adventurous. 'Betas,' by contrast, were lively, spontaneous, clever and flexible. The third category, the 'gammas' ... tended towards extremes -- sometimes they were overly cautious and self-deprecating, other times heedless and tyrannical ... Betz thinks temperaments may be the most important factor contributing to illness. 'It is the underlying core of the self,' she believes." (Newsweek, August 13, 1979, p. 40)

Ayurveda is more than a simple form of herbology. The vast literary tradition includes psychology, ontology and metaphysics. The great religious and scientific thinkers in Eastern medical history always stressed the development of mental faculties hand-in-hand with medical practice. Furthermore, Ayurveda is linked at all points with a responsible and ethical state of mind.

31

Ayurvedic Psychology

Practical help for the Vaidya to better understand patients' behavior is based on understanding the three major energies, nutritive, nervous and metabolic. According to Ayurvedic theory, one of these energies usually becomes dominant before birth and plays an important role in determining physical traits of the embryo. This, in turn, affects both the physiology and psychology of the person throughout his life. Ayurveda suggests three basic psycho-physiological types: **the nerve nature, the nutritive nature and the metabolic nature.** Experience shows about 60% of all people fall into one of these three basic types. The remaining 40% are mixed, usually having two dominant energies of about equal strength. The person with all three energies in equal balance is rare.

Both environmental and internal factors determine which energies and corresponding body systems will become dominant in each person. The condition of semen and ova, the diet and life regimen of the mother, the parents' age and psycho-physiological nature and so forth also contribute.

After birth the relative strengths of the body systems developing under the influence of the energies stabilize and do not change. For example, the person whose nutritive energy dominates, will have mucus membranes that are more sensitive and stronger in relationship to other body parts. These people will tend toward nutritive energy overbalance throughout their lives. The person whose metabolic energy is the strongest and most sensitive of the three will have relatively larger muscles, heart, veins, etc., and will have a tendency to metabolic energy overbalance. Similarly, the person whose nervous energy is the strongest will have a more sensitive brain and nerves than the other two types, and will be susceptible to nervous energy overbalance.

By studying the behavior and health of people from this reference, Ayurvedic concepts of balance and overbalance, and the relationship of physiology to personality can be understood. In our analysis, we will be generalizing and the considerable influence of family, environment, etc. will not be considered. All such factors can modify the basic psychophysiological character. And this is why Ayurvedic psychology, while simple in conception, becomes far from superficial in application.

DR. MANA: "In the beginning, I only had success treating nerve types. For me, the nerve-type Westerners are easy to handle. By nature, they are always sensitive, emotional and considerate. Whenever I diagnosed Western patients, they wanted to know how I came to conclusions about their condition. But they could not understand me when I tried to explain. My way did not make sense to them. Without understanding, it was difficult for them to accept my medicine. They usually understood herbal medicine was good, and they had confidence in the idea of natural cure, but when I would check their pulse, eyes, and so forth without modern equipment, they would question me. They especially could not understand how I could diagnose so quickly. I would try to explain, but it would take a long, long time, and I had to explain in many different ways. The nerve types, being naturally talkative and highly intelligent, would understand more quickly than the other types.

"Nutritive types are rare in Westerners. I had only a few of them, usually combined nature types (having two strong systems out of the major three). They also were easy, because they were accepting, gentle and kind. Most of the time, they didn't even ask why the medicine worked.

"However, I had considerable trouble with the metabolic types. Metabolic-type people are cautious by nature, and especially so with doctors because most of my patients have been treated unsuccessfully by Western doctors before coming to me. Metabolic-type people are aggressive and strong in body type, and they can quickly anger. For example, their type often gets fever. In the beginning stages of fever, it is difficult to determine the exact cause, and it takes time. The Ayurvedic approach is to give test medicine. If the patient immediately gets better, we continue the treatment; if not, we change the medicine. With metabolic types, if their fever does not immediately cease, they get irritated. By nature they demand instantaneous results. Also, they do not hesitate to try to dominate the doctor. The strong blood circulation is the cause of this because it can quickly become overbalanced. But, gradually, I learned how to deal with this type of patient"

The Nerve Nature

The person in whom the nervous energy is the strongest, most active and most sensitive of the three major energies is classified as a nerve-natured person. This type has a ten-dency to:

1. Be thin (See FIGURE 3).
When the nervous energy is more active, the nutritive energy is less active, causing a thinner, less well-nourished body. (See Page25)

2. Have large sense organs.
The sense organs are part of the nervous system, so they are larger than normal in a nerve-natured person.

3. Have thin skin with visible veins near the forehead.The minimal fat under the skin of nerve-natured people allows the veins to appear.

4. Have frequently changing facial expressions.
The nerve-natured person has quick mental and emotional reactions because of the nervous energy sensitivity. The eyes often dart quickly and the eyebrows raise.

Nerve-natured people, characteristically, display a great deal of cognitive intelligence or cleverness, and they are usually very talkative and friendly. In unfamiliar company or situations, however, they can be shy or reserved. They are prone to doubt and can change their minds incessantly under pressure. They are tentative, and this can affect their ability to carry out long-term goals. On the whole, they have scientific or logical minds, as well as active imaginations and enjoy the arts, sciences and literature.

The cognitive intelligence of nerve-natured people leads them to place great importance on personal understanding, while their physical sensitivity dictates the equal importance of personal safety, both physical and psychological. Because of this orientation, nerve-natured people are happiest when all personal and practical concerns are in harmony and balance, and least happy in moments of uncertainty or crisis.

Nerve-natured people often lead lives of constant and rapid change (e.g. change of job, change of friends etc.). They tend to be compassionate and willing, but are easily influenced by stronger personalities. They are often drawn to artistic or scholarly careers.

Nerve-natured people are more susceptible to nervous energy overbalance. Their physical structure is generally weaker than the other two types, and they often develop weak digestion, low immunity, strain in the lower back, legs and arms, slow circulation and joint pain. Their sensory organs deteriorate more rapidly than the other two types, and they often require glasses and hearing aids in later life.

The Metabolic Nature

The person in whom the metabolic energy is the strongest and most sensitive of the three major energies, is classified as metabolic natured. This type has a tendency to:

1. Be muscular (See FIGURE 2).
The strength of the metabolic energy increases digestive power, allowing the development of strong muscles.

2. Have forceful, sharp features and appearance.
The excess heat and energy generated by the strong metabolic energy contracts the features and creates an intensity of expression.

3. Perspire frequently or generate excess body heat.
The metabolic energy controls the body's thermogenic system, especially the dilation and contraction of capillaries. Being strong, it generates heat.

4. Highly energized and alert.
The metabolic energy provides plenty of energy for activity. Metabolic-natured people are highly individualistic, quick to react, both mentally and physically, and often require little sleep because of their excess energy. Their manner of speech is serious, and they tend to smile less than the other types. They enjoy adventurous and even dangerous activities, and do not hesitate to take risks. They are cautious without being fearful. These attributes lend themselves to success in business, politics and sports, especially in leadership positions.

Metabolic-natured people, because of their naturally high reserves of energy, often seek to maximize the energy, emotional and physical, in spite of possible consequences. Metabolic-natured people are happiest when they can be an

36

effective and unrestrained agent of change, and least happy when they are restricted in any way at all.

At times, metabolic-natured people can become aggressive or domineering and they quickly flare up and lose their tempers. They tend to become engrossed in their own ideas and interests which can annoy others. They tend to feel self-sufficient and that they can do it all themselves. This does not necessarily mean they are selfish, but only their awareness does not characteristically extend beyond their interests. As a result, they often disregard others unless there is a reason to include them. In other words, they use what is of value, and discard all else. Their extraordinary energy can make them valuable in anything they do. They require a firm foundation to properly channel their energy.

Metabolic-natured people are more susceptible to metabolic energy overbalance. They are prone to infections, high blood pressure and hyperacidity.

The Nutritive Nature
The person in whom the nutritive energy is the strongest, most active and most sensitive of the three major energies is classified as nutritive natured. These people tend to:

1. Have well-proportioned features (See FIGURE 6).
The nutritive energy relaxes the body, and keeps the facial features from contracting or being overactive.

2. Have a strong, robust and heavy body with a thick waist. The strong nutritive energy nourishes the body, causing it to become strong and heavy.

3. Have slow movement.
Because the nervous energy is less active when the nutritive energy is more active, the nutritive-natured person reacts and moves slowly.

37

4. Have soft watery eyes and a relaxed facial expression.
The strong nutritive system keeps the body well supplied with fluids.

5. Have thick, well-oiled skin.
Excess fat under the skin is a characteristic of nutritive-natured people.

Nutritive-natured people are relaxed, peaceful and content in their attitude and demeanor. They refuse to rush or hurry. Their speech is slow and they tend to have a broad and charming smile. They are usually compassionate and sociable, and reliable to carry out long-term projects and goals. Although they require lengthy deliberation before making up their minds, once they make the decision, they are extremely sure and deliberate in carrying it out. These characteristics lend themselves to success in the world.

Nutritive-natured people see life as nurturance and their central concern is to provide strength and stability to what is at hand. Nutritive-natured people are happiest when they can nurture and sustain in practical ways everything in their sphere of interest, including themselves. They are least happy when they can't do this.

Nutritive-natured people can be lethargic and dull if they are not in a balanced state of mental or physical health. They need to guard against long mental or emotional depressions. They enjoy study and can maintain a steady discipline, causing them to succeed where the quicker but less stable nerve-natured person might fail. Nutritive-natured people often are sought as counselors because they listen well and can easily empathize with others' concerns. They require little of others and pose no threat. They often become professional planners or organizers of groups of people.

Nutritive-natured people are prone to nutritive energy over-balance. Because of their bodies' strength and solidity, they often exhibit good health throughout life. When they become sick, it is usually with respiratory problems, asthma, allergies, obesity, swelling, coughs and colds.

To correctly determine the three natures requires skill. A teacher's guidance is often needed because the determination is made on a preponderance of characteristics, rather than a single one. For example, sometimes nerve-natured people are heavy (See Page 34), and nutritive-natured people thin (See Page 37). The heaviness of the nerve-natured person, however, will differ from the nutritive-natured person to the trained eye. Metabolic-natured people may appear gentle or smile often (See Page 36), as might be the case of a metabolic-natured person who is highly educated. All such characteristics must be allowed in analysis.

It is possible to see the three natures in terms of geographical influences. India, for example, has a higher than normal percentage of nerve-natured people, while Germany has a higher percentage of metabolic-natured people. The United States, on the other hand, has a lesser amount of nutritive-natured people. This is because of environmental and dietary conditions affecting the mothers before and during pregnancy.

When the person's nature is difficult to determine, the best procedure is to eliminate one of the three types. For example, if a person seems to have both nerve and metabolic char-acteristics, but lacks nutritive characteristics, he should be classified as nerve-metabolic natured.

	Nutritive Nature	Metabolic Nature	Nerve Nature
Eyes	peaceful, watery	forceful, glaring	moving, darting
Mouth	broad smile	stern, few smiles	frequent smile
Body	strong, heavy	muscular, warm	thin, cold
Speech	low, peaceful	serious	rapid, changeable

Figure 6. Identifying characteristics of the three natures.

Practical Applications

The Ayurvedic Vaidya must determine his patient's nature at a glance. Each nature has a characteristic way of acting and reacting. Knowing the patient's nature gives the Vaidya important information about the person's physical condition. Nerve-natured people tend to be weaker and develop nervous energy overbalance; metabolic-natured people tend to be aggressive and develop metabolic energy overbalance, and nutritive-natured people tend to be strong and develop nutritive energy overbalance.

The Vaidya will establish rapport with his patient by mirroring his nature. That is, he will be talkative and friendly with a nerve-natured patient, easygoing and compassionate with a nutritive-natured patient, and energetic and forceful with a metabolic-natured patient. This approach is extremely effective in the initial stages of interaction because the patient will feel secure and understood by the doctor who shares his psychological pattern. This is, however, only a starting point in the relationship. The Vaidya's ultimate goal is to deal with his patients in a gentle, nurturing, yet effective manner. Generally speaking, nerve and nutritive-natured patients are easy to manage, while metabolic-natured patients are often more difficult because of their tendency to want to dominate or control relationships.

The Meaning of Life

The nature of life, mind and body are necessarily abstract. Ayurveda's history extends thousands of years and embraces countless metaphysical positions from its diverse religious and cultural background. It is characteristic of nations and cultures, religious groups and even families, no less than scientific disciplines, to claim purity of lineage. In this section we will present a Buddhist school of Ayurvedic thought about the meaning of life, mind and body, without claiming there are no other lines of thought with equal claims to validity. The Buddhists emphasize that their ideas are consistent in their major lineaments with the positions presented first in the *Charaka Samhita* and the *Susruta Samhita,* although they deny the necessity of including Atma (soul or Self) in their definition of life. (The Hindu schools include Atma.)

To understand the Ayurvedic concept of life, we must expand the use of the abstract metaphysical principles of creation, destruction and order. In the first chapter we defined "body" as the interplay of these three principles, or from a purely physical view. From a different and large perspective, we can use these principles as means of understanding body, mind and life. For example, the creative principle is mind, while the destructive principle is body. The mind is unitary and whole, creating and sustaining the created; the body and the physical universe are diverse, and always decaying or being destroyed. In this formula, the mind has a logical priority over the body; the body exists within and under the direction of the mind. It is, however, impossible to separate mind and body in understanding either, and it is an over-simplification to identify mind as not-body and body as not-mind. These two are different sides of the same coin, so to speak. The body is the polar complement of the mind which creates and sustains it.[17]

Life is the merging of these two principles in a universe of constant change. Life is that which exists between creation and

41

destruction, or mind and body. The dynamic principle of order integrates them. The Ayurvedic idea of life as an integrating principle between mind and body frees it from its attachment only to the physical organism. This is clear by its identification in Sanskrit as prana or life current. Prana is life as a universal current or stream flowing between mind and body. Both mental and physical, it is known through its effect on the regulation of the brain's mental and sensory processes, and on organic vitality. In higher states of consciousness it is possible to experience directly. Prana, and its five divisions in the body according to function, is a higher ordering of the nervous energy, which controls its flow through the body.

The mind and body counterreact with each other through prana. The mental activates the physical and the physical activates the mental. In other words, a positive state of mind helps energize the body, and a positive state of health helps energize and clear the mind. The first half of this is known in Western psychology as the placebo effect, but the Eastern view is without negative connotations. The Ayurvedic Vaidya tries to inspire the patient to have confidence in his medicine and treatment. To him, this is transferring his mental energy or confidence to the patient's mind, so it can activate the physical medicine. Without confidence, the medicine will be less effective. This can't be overstressed. The degree to which the mind and body counterreact positively with each other affects the flow of prana, and can be measured by the coordination within the nervous system and overall vitality.

Faculties of Mind
The sense organs concentrate the mind for perception. As the brain, almost a sixth sense which perceives the mind, organizes sense data and thoughts into concepts, words and language to be referred to the mind for understanding, the individual reacts to the world. Normally, he will enjoy and be attracted to whatever brings him happiness and fulfillment, and will reject whatever brings suffering. This is the Ayurvedic concept of the well-integrated person.

When the individual can't function this way -- when he is drawn to what brings suffering and rejects what brings happiness -- he is in an unhealthy state of mind. When this occurs, it can be traced to a deficiency in the natural flowering of one or more of the eight faculties of mind described by Ayurveda. These are:

1. Understanding
Understanding is the ability to correlate ordinary, sense-derived knowledge with an intuitive perception of the fundamental principles of the universe (or nature). Understanding can be developed through spiritual practice or meditation and because this faculty of mind allows the development of creative mental competence, it is of high importance.

2. Consciousness
Consciousness is the measure of the ability to receive and coordinate mental input, and it defines the scope of perceived reality. A properly functioning consciousness can coordinate the impulses from the senses and memory in a way leading to happiness and fruitful action. An improperly functioning consciousness will be uncoordinated and distracted, just as when someone looks at a scene without understanding or eats something without being aware of tasting it.

3. Memory
Memory is the record of past understanding and experience. Whatever is well understood remains in memory a long time. Whatever is poorly understood fades quickly. Memory controls desire because positive or negative feelings associated with a recorded memory create anticipation of future events.

4. Thinking
Thinking is the faculty of mind at work when it is not focused on present sense perceptions or higher mental functions, such as meditation, but is focused on the memories. Thinking can be positive or negative, depending on how it is used. If it is

habitual and unproductive, it is negative. If it is controlled and useful it is positive.

5. Preference
The mind quickly develops preferences with regard to colors, sounds, ideologies and so forth. Preferences change and become less mechanical as the other faculties develop.

6. Natural Tendency
Natural tendencies are mental characteristics held from birth such as sensitivity, aggressiveness, boldness and indifference, and can be deduced from understanding the three natures. Natural tendencies can be altered by developing the mental faculties.

7. Emotion
Emotions express the immediate tenor of mind and, as such, color all other faculties. Emotions are clearly defined by Ayurveda according to changes in facial expressions and subtle hues from the skin. For example, eyes wide open and bulging from excess blood volume in the head indicate the physical correlation to anger. Nine emotions are counted: anger, love, laughter, compassion, bravery, dreadfulness, disgust, wonder and peacefulness.

8. Discipline
Discipline as a faculty of mind refers to an individual's ability to conform to order or structure, or to an inwardly held goal or purpose.

States of Mind
The eight faculties of mind are tools for measuring mind-body integration. Their development or non-development and their use creates the individual state of mind. Ayurveda recognizes three states of mind: the pure mind, the aggressive mind and the indolent mind (sattvic, rajasic and tamasic). The person with a pure mind has developed the eight faculties. He is free of attachments, fully conscious and highly moral. The

44

person with the aggressive mind has developed faculties of mind, but neglected understanding or lost control of natural tendencies or preferences. The person with the indolent mind neglected to develop his faculties of mind to any appreciable extent.

The attributes of a person in any of these three states are described in clear-cut terms. Of course, one's "state of mind" is a complex continuum, everyone can be in a pure, an aggressive or an indolent state of mind at different times. An individual is categorized in a particular state of mind because he characteristically thinks and acts according to that type.

The Pure State of Mind

People with pure states of mind may have quite distinct personalities, and may come from totally different backgrounds, training and cultures. These people display:

1. Orderliness and cleanliness
The mind when properly functioning through the body demands orderliness. The pure mind is one in which the memories and thoughts are always in order, like a well-kept filing cabinet. This is reflected externally by cleanliness in personal habits and an orderly lifestyle.

2. Truthfulness
The mind knows the homogeneousness and worth of all human beings. Therefore, it is not intent upon the survival of its goals at the expense of others, it considers the needs of others as its own. It is not afraid of facts and, thus, has no reason to distort the truth.

3. Balance
The pure mind is, by nature, balanced. It does not have imbalancing sensory cravings, delusions, hatred, so forth.

4. Gentleness and harmlessness
The individual can do no harm because he sees others as a part of himself. Harming others clearly creates confusion and loss of peace of mind. This does not mean weakness and apathy; the person can handle his affairs firmly.

5. Trustworthiness
The smooth working of society depends upon respecting the rules and customs of the majority. Realizing this, the person of pure mind is trustworthy and reliable.

6. Intelligence
The pure state of mind is often described in the Ayurvedic literature as crystalline in clarity. It resembles a jewel of many facets, and is capable and efficient. It has naturally quick understanding, clear judgment, desire for true knowledge, keen memory and realization of the true cause and effect.

7. Sensitivity
This person is sensitive to the realities of others. He includes rather than excludes others from his sensitivity.

8. Open-mindedness
To be open-minded is to be free from fixation to a particular view, while remaining faithful to one's principles. The individual grows through openness to new experience and learning.

The Aggressive State of Mind
The aggressive mind is in individuals who lost their understanding of the mind's unitary nature. In Western terms they have an egotistical or self-centered point of view. They are unaware of their connection to all other sentient beings. Such people are survival-oriented as opposed to altruistic. These people display:

1. Aggressiveness
The person is fearful and hostile and sees himself competing with the rest of the world.

2. Untrustworthiness
The person sees no advantage to obeying rules or conforming to the dictates of society, except as it serves his ends.

3. Addictiveness
The person has sensory imbalance. Sensory gratifications provide escapes from pain. These people are easily addicted to indulgence in food, alcohol, sex, luxuries and so forth.

4. Selfishness
The person is obsessed with their self-importance. His personal needs are paramount.

The Indolent State of Mind
The indolent-mind person has lost his sense of purpose. This comes from neglecting to develop the eight faculties of the mind. As a result, there is little awareness beyond immediate survival. These people display:

1. Laziness
The person is actually semi-conscious and will very easily withdraw into sleep and lethargy.

2. Indulgence
When the person shows some movement or initiative, he is interested only in food, sex, alcohol, etc. He shares this characteristic with aggressive-minded people.

3. Stupidity
The person can't properly assess or arrange mental input.

Mental Illness
Usually, mental illness occurs because of one of the two unhealthy states of mind. The aggressive-mind person is in

47

danger of succumbing to anger or negative emotions, which weaken the nervous energy system and its coordination. The indolent-mind person is in danger of entering delusional states, which also creates coordination loss in the nervous system. This lack of coordination upsets the person's ability to react properly.

Physical problems also can cause mental illness, but less often. For example, a pregnant woman who is sick or leads an unhealthy life can give birth to children with mental problems. In such cases, Ayurveda treats the patient according to the physical balance theory.

Mental patients display loss of coordination in their nervous system and negative emotions. The Vaidya must distinguish between the emotions and the forms of lack of coordination before treatment. This is done by watching the body's physical movements and gestures and sense organs, and changes in skin hues or superficial circulation. This requires knowing the flow of nerve currents and prana. For example, patients may appear to be crying while they are laughing, with their mouths turned down and eyes constricted during the laugh.

There are two major treatment approaches to mental disorder: meditation and ritual practice, and emotional counter-reaction. Meditation/ritual practice relaxes the patient and restores balance to the sense organs. The patient might be sent to a quiet and peaceful environment, such as temple, and instructed to do religious chanting, prayer and so forth.

Emotional counterreaction neutralizes negative emotions rooted in the patient's mind. Emotions are paired in opposites (which can overlap). Lust counteracts anger, for example, and anger counteracts fear. So if the patient exhibits uncontrollable anger, sexual activity might be prescribed to neutralize the fear. The use of this treatment requires much practice.

Summary

Ayurvedic psychology is based on interpreting physical and personality traits in terms of the three major energy systems. The person with a strong nervous energy is considered nerve natured. He will be thin and nervous, with quick mental and physical reactions. The person with a strong metabolic energy is considered metabolic natured. He will be muscular and alert, with a powerful individualistic personality, sometimes dom-inating. The person with a strong nutritive energy is con-sidered nutritive natured. He will be heavy and peaceful looking, with a calm, relaxed personality, sometimes tending to lethargy. The Vaidya uses this knowledge to deal with his patients effectively, both psychologically and physically.

The principles of creation, destruction and order can be used to delineate mind, body and life, respectively. Life means the merging of mind into body and vice versa. The concept of life is extended to mean an unceasing flow of prana, or life current, between mind and body. In the individual, life current is seen in the coordination of concepts and mental states. This can be measured by the degree of development of the eight faculties of mind: understanding, consciousness, memory, thinking, preference, natural tendency, emotion and discipline.

The mind and body counterreact. Mental energy is necessary to activate physical energy. The Vaidya stimulates confidence in the patient's mind to increase the medicine's effectiveness. As opposed to the pure state of mind, there are two negative states: the aggressive and indolent minds. Both states lead to a loss of coordination in the nervous system, with a decrease in physical and mental well-being. There are two major treatments to mental disorder: meditation to restore balance to the sense organs and the nervous energy; and emotional counterreaction to neutralize strong negative emo-tional states.

Part Two

The Practical Basis of Ayurveda

Tillotson: "I am wondering why Ayurveda has remained so small and unknown outside India and Nepal in spite of its successful treatments and long history? The government doesn't seem to support you, and some Nepalis seem to prefer Western medicine."

Dr. Mana: "Very good, Alan. This is the question I want to be asked, the question I want to answer.

"The first thing you have to know is that almost all Ayurvedic books are written in Sanskrit. The knowledge and study of Ayurveda is limited to those who know Sanskrit. This is the first big problem. To have Westerners learn Ayurveda would require the translation of all the texts into English. This is why I am writing books in English.

"Also, there is politics involved. I have been teaching Ayurveda to Westerners for a long time. But whenever these people go back to their countries, they cannot practice even simple cures; it is illegal. In your country the rule of the A.M.A. (American Medical Association) does not allow any other doctors to practice in any case. We allow them to practice here, but they do not allow us to practice. This is politics. From my point of view, the new generation has to change the law.

"Of course, many M.D.s are interested in Ayurveda, and they can practice it if they learn it. But this is very limited. I am making a big effort to talk with them and involve them. I would like them to join with us and create a more holistic medicine in the world. There are so many diseases which we Ayurvedic doctors can cure which our Western friends can't.

"If they want proof, I invite them to come to my clinic here. They can see, obviously, whether I can cure or not. But the prejudice, so far, has not allowed them to accept Ayurveda.

"The scientific principles of Ayurveda are completely different from those of Western medicine. They are not based upon the germ theory. They are based on the balance theory - the balance of the physical body. Ayurvedic doctors accept the existence of germs because, obviously, we can see them. We know they exist. However, we don't use this theory for treatment. Without antibiotic treatment my patients get better in three or four days from amoebic dysentery, Giardia, bacillary dysentery, and so forth. This is difficult for the mind to accept if it is only thinking of germs.

"Economics is also involved. In the West, there are big, big pharmaceutical companies which have a monopoly on medicine. Medicine is big business. They don't want other medicines to compete with them. In my country there are some allopathic (Western contemporary medicine) hospitals and health clinics. Western pharmaceutical companies are supporting them, and they offer free medicine and free treatment for Nepalis. Many city people go to these hospitals; the poor people are especially allured. But the Ayurvedic doctors cannot give free medicine. We do not have even a single rupee in aid. Even so, I tell you that most of the people in my country are not interested in allopathic medicine. Only a small percentage go to the clinics. Some of the rich Nepalis go to the hospitals because they have been strongly influenced by Western culture.

"I don't want you to think I am talking with pride -- saying that Ayurveda is better than anything else, or that it can cure everything. There is no doubt that Ayurveda is an effective medicine. However, it must be prescribed with education, knowledge and understanding. If people use it improperly, they will not have success. To use Ayurveda properly, you must know the exact condition of overbalance in the body. Many bad or untrained doctors in the past and even now have hurt the reputation of Ayurveda. Of the hundreds of Ayurvedic doctors in my country, only a few have been properly trained. Many of them have lost faith from not having any support. This is not the government's fault -- they do not have money for aid. Is it clear to you now why Ayurveda has not spread to other parts of the world?"

Chapter Three
Diagnosis

"Edgar Cayce, in looking at the sickness of the human bodies that were presented to him for clairvoyant commentary, seemed to find within these individuals a variety of incoordinations. He found this so consistently that we are forced to attempt an understanding of what he described so often as incoordination, and what we think of as being basically a lack of balance."

William A. McGarey, M.D.
Director, Association for Research and
Enlightenment Clinic
Phoenix, Ariz.

We introduced the Ayurvedic concept of disease -- the result of overbalance of one or more of the three major energy systems. Ayurvedic diagnosis identifies the major factors that overbalance each energy system and the ways to assess this overbalance. To accomplish this, diagnosis is divided into five sections:

1. The causes of disease
2. Precursor symptomatology
3. Symptoms
4. Morbid anatomy in diseases
5. Testing

The Causes of Disease

To understand how Ayurveda determines the factors overbalancing any one of the three major energy systems, it is necessary to understand the concept of samanya (See Page 62). Samanya means the affinity of similar objects, properties and energies for each other. In practical terms, this means nervous energy, for example, is light, fine, dry and movable in its properties, and being an electric or vibratory type of energy, will be increased by anything with similar properties or energy entering the body. This includes all sorts of physical, light and sound vibrations. All influences affect a system in proportion to the degree of similarity. Metabolic energy, for instance, is strongly affected by heat, both internal and external, because it is hot in property. This is samanya.

In many ways, this is a common sense way of understanding experience. It is obvious that nervousness is increased by loud sounds and noises, and nourishment is enhanced when we eat in a calm and restful atmosphere. We say the loud sounds and noises disturb us and the calm atmosphere relaxes us, but we would be hard put to explain why. Here, Ayurveda presents a simple yet effective explanation. Loud vibrations share qualities with nervous energy, and this input affects it more than the other two energy systems. Similarly, a calm and restful atmosphere shares qualities with nutritive energy, and enhances it more than the other two energy systems. All phenomena are related to their effects on the three primary energies through samanya.

Nervous Energy Overbalance

Nervous energy has the physical properties of being light, dry, cold, movable, fine, non-viscous, and harsh; and electrical or vibratory in nature. By using samanya we can discover the internal and external factors that might cause overbalance to the point of disease.

Stress affects nervous energy strongly and we can see this in someone under stress. Eyes dart around quickly, body movements become shaky or uncoordinated, and thinking becomes unclear. The stressful conditions elicit perceptions of possible future events that conflict with the reality of ideas, concepts, memories, and hopes which nervous energy regulates. In other words, nervous energy causes us to anticipate

54

danger or unpleasant events and to react. These perceptions share properties of nervous energy; they are light, fine, and electrical or vibratory; thus fear, hyperactivity and nervousness all relate to what Ayurveda calls nervous energy overbalance.

Certain physical and sensory trauma also affect nervous energy, such as the vibrations of riding in trucks or buses, or of being near large, noisy machines. Another example is overfocusing on things which strongly stimulate the sense organs. This includes watching too much television, listening to loud or discordant sounds for long times, staring at bright lights, etc. These influences are all light, fine and vibratory.

Nutrition is a third major factor affecting nervous energy directly. In this case, the analysis is a little different. Ayurveda first analyzes foods for their tastes and uses this analysis to determine the physical properties (See Chapter 5). Bitter, pungent and astringent foods affect nervous energy strongly because they are light, fine, dry, etc. in physical property. This is a complicated subject and there are many exceptions. Besides taste, cold can overbalance nervous energy, e.g., too much ice cream or cold drinks.

Other factors include cold weather, which causes trembling and shaking and lack of sleep, without which nervous energy cannot restore itself. Nervous energy regulates the movement of blood, stool, urine, etc., throughout the body and anything interfering with these processes overbalances it. Loss of blood, for example, or suppressing natural urges (gas, stool, urine) can have this result.

Of course, many other factors affect nervous energy. This brief list, however, should illustrate the reasoning Ayurveda employs to determine effects of different phenomena on nervous energy.

Metabolic Energy Overbalance

Metabolic energy has the physical properties of being hot, oily, penetrating, movable and liquid. It is quite changeable and will be quickly affected by anything having similar properties. Hot liquids quickly affect metabolic energy, as do fast-penetrating acid foods. Again, this is a generalization; other factors, such as chemical actions, food preparation and so forth can be inhibiting or releasing factors.

Anger and similar powerful emotions quickly upset and overbalance metabolic energy, just as stress overbalances nervous energy. An angry person literally becomes hot and red-faced, with bulging eyes and all these are symptoms of metabolic overbalance.

Heat is an important factor. Smoking, working in excess heat and overexposure to the sun heat the body, which stimulates metabolic energy. Too much leads to overbalance. Similarly, acid-forming or pungent (hot) foods vigorously stimulate metabolic energy. This includes coffee, tea, meat, alcohol, sour fruit, vinegar, and hot spices. Practical experimentation with diet can demonstrate this.

Nutritive Energy Overbalance

Nutritive energy is cold, soft, oily, solid, viscous and heavy. This energy is peaceful, nourishing and strengthening. Nutritive energy quickly responds to anything with similar properties, increasing its activities. For example, oily and heavy foods may cause nutritive energy overbalance.

In contrast to the causes of nervous energy overbalance, nutritive energy can become overbalanced through lethargy. Emotional withdrawal, indifference and apathy cause nutritive energy overbalance, as does oversleeping, sleeping during the day or living in a dull or unstimulating atmosphere. Because nutritive energy controls absorption of food, the result is often overeating.

Nutritive energy controls absorption of air and water, as well as food. So polluted water and air can cause overbalance. Heavy, oily and difficult to digest foods also cause over-balance, as do milk products.

These and similar factors are considered primary causes of major energy overbalances. Studying these causes through inductive logic and observation is an integral part of Ayurvedic diagnosis. Mental and emotional states, personal behavior and diet are direct causes of disease, and personal responsibility in shaping these plays an important part in Ayurvedic therapy.

Secondary Causes of Disease

Ayurveda generally describes disease as occurring through: (primary cause -> overbalance of major energy -> disease). However, specific secondary causes are linked with certain diseases without reference to overbalance of energy systems. This would be: (secondary cause -> disease).

Some examples are:
1. Certain clays in food that cause anemia
2. Excess iron in the diet that causes gallstones
3. Mica in the diet that causes liver pain
4. Copper in the diet that causes vomiting
5. Ear wax that causes migraine headaches
6. Pollen that causes hay fever
7. Lead contamination that causes joint pain

Ayurvedic texts also mention germs and parasites found in blood, stool, mucus or skin. A number of these are described in detail, along with specific habits or practices which allow them to develop. Thus:

1. Pathogenic bacteria in the blood develop through therm-ogenic imbalance, indigestion, eating antagonistic foods (See Chapter 5) and, especially, poor diet. In general, they are responsible for infections, eczema, scabies and other con-ditions.

57

2. There are five major categories of parasites which live in the stool. They are the result of improper diet, eating rotten or decayed foods, and indigestion. And they cause diarrhea, constipation, colic, itching of the anus, goose pimples and weight loss, etc. If parasites reach the stomach, the result is stomach distress, belching and burping.

3. Seven major categories of parasites live in mucus. These usually originate in the stomach and spread through the body. They develop because of improper diet, indigestion, eating rotten or decayed foods, etc. Some are white and flat, some are pink and worm-like, and some are quite small and fiber-like. They can cause nausea, fever, body ache, sneezing, vomiting, bloated stomach and loss of weight and appetite.

Besides these, Ayurveda recognizes countless pathogenic bacteria. Epidemics and extremely contagious diseases -- which are characterized by the sudden appearance of symptoms without indication of major system overbalance -- are caused by these bacteria. Such diseases include cholera, tetanus, meningitis and encephalitis. These diseases are called in Sanskrit "grahadoshas", meaning "celestial diseases" -- diseases of the air and water. Many children's diseases are in this category. Historically, because of their virulence, these diseases were in the spiritual healing division of Ayurveda.

The three categories of parasites then cause diseases along the pattern of (improper behavior -> overbalance of major energy -> multiplication of parasites -> diseases). The more virulent bacteria, however, can cause disease directly along the pattern of (infiltration of bacteria from polluted air or water - > disease). That is to say, even a healthy person is susceptible to disease if he is living in an environment of polluted air or water.

A final cause of disease is another disease, according to Ayurveda. A coronary, for example, can lead to breathlessness or cough; anemia can lead to heart disease or hepatitis; chronic influenza can lead to tuberculosis, and gout can lead to cancer.

Knowing these causes is very important and a Vaidya must identify these secondary diseases when taking a case history. Where anemia leads to hepatitis, for example, both conditions must be simultaneously treated for a cure, by treating metabolic energy overbalance and the specific symptoms of anemia and hepatitis.

Precursor Symptoms

When one of the three major energy systems is overbalanced, the body can't carry out its normal activities. In this state, the body creates toxins. If nutritive energy is overbalanced, the body will secrete toxic or salty mucus. If the nervous energy is overbalanced, the body creates putrefactive gases. For example, in hepatitis, the bile duct is blocked. Then nervous energy cannot direct bile to the intestines and food rots there, giving off putrefactive gases. Any time the nervous energy is too overbalanced to cause the circulation of fluids, blood, lymph, etc., these will decompose in the body and give off gases. If metabolic energy is overbalanced, various acid toxins or "sour bile" will result. These categories of toxins - salty mucus, putrefactive gases and sour bile - then circulate through the body, causing precursor symptoms. When toxins settle in an organ or system, they cause morbidity and the appearance of true disease symptoms. Examples of precursor symptoms are:

1. Fatigue, uneasiness, watery eyes, yawning, body ache, goose pimples and loss of appetite are the precursors of fever. They are caused by circulating "sour bile".

2. Rapid onset of constipation, bloated stomach, abdominal pain and indigestion are the precursors of diarrhea. They are caused by putrefactive gases.

3. A sweet taste in the mouth, hot sensation in the feet and hands, oily skin, thirst and a white coating in the teeth are precursors of diabetes. They are caused by circulating "sour bile" and undigested sugar.

General Symptoms of Major Energy Overbalance

When any energy system becomes overbalanced it will exhibit certain general symptoms. Of course, there will be additional symptoms characteristic of that disease.

When nervous energy is dominating, the usual symptoms are:

1. Sharp local pain, decreasing with application of pressure
2. Throbbing pain
3. Colic
4. Dryness
5. Weak or slowed circulation
6. Numbness
7. Nervous movement
8. Emaciation
9. Malaise
10. Blue or pink coloration in the affected area, often spreading to complexion, urine, stool, eyes and tongue.

When nutritive energy is dominating, the usual symptoms are:

1. Mild local pain, unaffected by the application of pressure
2. Itching
3. Blocked internal ducts
4. Slow circulation
5. Abnormal growth
6. Overexudation of mucus
7. Swelling
8. Slowed responses to stimuli
9. White or pale coloration in the affected area, often spreading to the complexion, urine, stool, eyes or tongue.

When metabolic energy is dominating, the usual symptoms are:
1. Burning local pain, made worse when applying pressure
2. Inflammation

3. Infection
4. Fever
5. Hot flashes
6. Blood discharge, rapid decay
7. Strong body odor
8. Fatigue
9. Yellow or red coloration in the affected area, often spreading to the complexion, urine, stool, eyes or tongue

These general symptoms may be very clear or very subtle, but they give the Vaidya valuable information on the disease's cause. Many diseases are common to certain energy groups. Hypoglycemia, for example, is classified as a nerve energy disease, not only because of the symptoms, but also because it affects a high percentage of nerve-natured people. Metabolic-natured people, on the other hand, will have a greater chance of heart attacks (cf. modern research on Type A and Type B heart attack proclivity).

Study of Morbid Anatomy
Morbid anatomy is the detailed analysis of sick organs or body systems. Diseased organs are examined to determine if size, location and degree of functioning is normal. For example, in hepatitis, the liver is enlarged. When examined, the patient experiences tenderness or sharp pain from applied pressure and during inhalation will feel more pain. Swelling and mucus cause the billiary duct to close, causing the bile produced by the liver to flow back into the blood circulation. This study is very thorough in Ayurveda. Special attention is given to arterial supply of nutrients (Kapha), venous drainage of metabolic by-products (Pitta) and nerve and prana supply (Vata) (See FIGURE 4, Chapter Two).

Testing
It is very important to correctly diagnose which energy system is overbalanced and to what degree. In complicated and unclear cases, medicines and diet may be given to aggravate or subdue the condition and test for the cause. For example, in

61

colic pain it is often unclear which major energy is over-balanced. It might be the nervous or the nutritive energies. In such a case, the Vaidya will give foods and medicines to stimulate the nutritive energy. If the patient gets worse, this indicates the colic is caused by overbalanced nervous energy and stimulating nutritive energy restores balance (according to the formula: nervous energy <-> nutritive energy).

In addition to determining the primary cause of disease, checking precursor symptoms, symptoms, morbid anatomy and testing to clarify the determination, Ayurvedic Vaidyas also test pulse, eye color, tongue, stool, urine, etc. and take case histories.

With regard to the pulse, Ayurveda explains that nervous energy overbalances always present a thin, fleeting pulse; metabolic energy overbalances present a fast, strongly bounding or jumping pulse, and nutritive energy overbalances present soggy, dull impulses which rebound from the upper to the lower surfaces of the artery.

In taking case histories, Ayurvedic Vaidyas attempt to understand the progression of the condition. This is crucial in complicated cases. For example, in cases of joint pain, patients with histories of gout, rheumatism and gas problems would be diagnosed as arthritic, whereas, if there was no such history, joint pain would probably be considered the result of injury.

Summary
Ayurveda uses the concept of samanya -- the affinity of similar objects, properties and energies, and their tendency to assimilate into each other -- to determine what overbalances the three major energy systems. Nervous energy is light, dry, cold, movable, fine, non-viscous and harsh in physical property, and electrical or vibratory in nature. It can be overbalanced by stress, overstimulation of sense organs, discordant vibrations, bitter, pungent and astringent foods, cold weather and suppression of natural bodily urges.

Metabolic energy is hot, oily, penetrating, movable and liquid in physical property and changeable. It can be overbalanced by anger, powerful emotions, heat, and acidic or pungent foods. Nutritive energy is cold, soft, oily, solid, viscous and heavy in physical property, and nourishing and strengthening in nature. It can be overbalanced by lethargy, oversleeping, polluted air or water, heavy and oily foods, and milk products. Certain things -- such as lead or clay in the diet -- can cause disease before overbalancing one of three major energies. Very strong bacteria from polluted air or water also can directly cause disease. An untreated disease can cause another disease.

When the nutritive energy is overbalanced, the body secretes toxic or "salty" mucus. When metabolic energy is overbalanced, the body creates acidic toxins or "sour bile". When the nervous energy is overbalanced, the body cannot circulate substances and fluids, causing putrefactive gases. These toxins move through the body causing precursor symptoms. When nervous energy is overbalanced, the major symptoms are pain, dryness and nervous movement. When metabolic energy is overbalanced, major symptoms are burning pain, fever, excess heat and fatigue. When nutritive energy is overbalanced, the major symptoms are over-exudation of mucus, blocked internal ducts and lethargy. Ayurvedic Vaidyas make detailed studies of morbid anatomy and case histories. In complicated cases, test medicines are given to clarify conditions.

Chapter Four

Pharmacology and Medicinal Plants

"Long before we discovered their use in the West, traditional Indian physicians were using such preparations as reserpine to lower blood pressure and calm nerves, cardia glycosides similar to digitalis to regulate the rhythm of the heart, and fungal preparations similar to penicillin as antibiotics."

Rudolph Ballentine, M.D.
Director of the Combined Therapy Clinic
Himalayan Institute
Honesdale, PA.

Ayurvedic pharmacology is unique in classifying medicines. Empirical testing and sharpened sensory awareness skills iso-late the factors governing the activity of medicines. All herbs, medicines and foods are analyzed according to the medicines.

1. Activity classified by taste
2. Physical properties
3. Heating and cooling properties
4. Actions affected by digestion
5. Specific actions

The Sense of Taste

Ayurvedic Vaidyas primarily use their taste sense to determine the pharmacological properties of foods and medicines. Just as an artist must know the primary colors, the Vaidya must know the six basic tastes: sweet, sour, salty, bitter, pungent and astringent. Western physiology also recognizes that the sense of taste has an amazing degree of discrimination, often out-doing modern technological equipment in detecting subtle factors. The range of sensitivity required of Ayurvedic Vaidyas seems astounding. Sixty-four combinations of the six basic tastes were recorded and used in the ancient texts of Ayurvedic medicine.

According to Ayurvedic theory, a medicine's taste shows how it will affect the body. A Vaidya trained to use his sense of taste can determine whether a medicine will speed or slow the heart, constrict or dilate the capillaries, increase or decrease mucus and so forth -- by taste alone. Of course, the most important use of this information is to determine the medicine's effects on the three major energies.

To use taste, a student learns to differentiate the six basic tastes and their physical effects on the body. This list shows each taste with familiar foods exemplifying them.

1. Sweet
Sweet-tasting foods nourish the body, and this taste is the most abundant. Sweet-tasting foods are: rice, wheat, barley, meat, milk, cream, sugar, cheese, eggs, honey, etc. These foods help increase the body constituents, such as flesh and fat, neutralize toxins; heal and replace tissues, and increase weight. They primarily stimulate nutritive energy.

2. Sour
Among the sour-tasting foods are: lemon, lime, tomato, yogurt and vinegar. The sour foods increase appetite, dissolve foods to promote digestion, regulate peristaltic movement in the alimentary system and stimulate the internal organs, especially the heart. They also increase weight and strength. Sour foods and medicines stimulate metabolic and nutritive energies.

3. Salty
Salt increases the appetite and aids blood circulation and digestion through its ability to dissolve. In addition, salt increases thirst and water retention in the body. Salty foods and medicines stimulate the metabolic and nutritive energies.

4. Bitter
Bitter taste is primarily in foods and spices such as: tumeric, fenugreek, cumin seeds, mace, parsley, coffee and most teas. The bitter taste increases the appetite, regulates body temperature, helps maintain skin moisture, aids fat metabolism and cleanses the blood. In general, it is purifying. Bitter foods and medicines stimulate nervous energy.

5. Pungent
Pungent or hot taste is in spices such as cayenne, black pepper, ginger and garlic. Their heating effect increases the appetite, stops overexudation of mucus and abnormal growth, and cleanses the duct systems by breaking up blockages of mucus and coagulated blood. Pungent foods and medicines stimulate the metabolic and nervous energies.

6. Astringent
The astringent taste in foods causes the mucus membranes and other tissues to shrink and draw together. Astringency is tissue strengthening. The effect is drying to the body. This "taste" is really an effect found in combination with other tastes (e.g. sweet-astringent or sour-astringent). It is in all beans, honey and unripe fruit. Astringent foods and medicines strengthen capillaries and red blood cells, solidify the stool and help regulate bile production. They stimulate nervous energy.

The Physical Properties of Medicines
A corollary use of taste is to determine the physical properties of foods and medicines. Ayurveda lists 10 pairs of such physical properties:

1. Heavy to digest - Light to digest

2. Oily - Drying
3. Heating - Cooling
4. Softening - Hardening
5. Viscous - Non-viscous
6. Movement increasing - Movement decreasing
7. Smooth - Harsh
8. Mild (slow acting) - Strong (quick acting)
9. Liquid - Solid
10. Fine - Coarse

The first three pairs are the most important in pharmacology because they strongly affect the major energies. Medicines that are oily or heavy to digest will strongly stimulate nutritive energy. Medicines that are drying or light to digest will strongly stimulate nervous energy. Heating and cooling medicines affect metabolic energy.

The physical properties of medicines usually correlate very well with the six tastes. It's important to know the many exceptions to this classification system.

| | | Major Energy Stimulated | | |
Taste	Keyword	Nervous	Metabolic	Nutritive
Sweet	Nourishing			X
Sour	Stimulating		X	
Salty	Dissolving		X	X
Bitter	Purifying	X		
Pungent	Heating	X	X	
Astringent	Drying	X		

FIGURE 7 The effects of the six tastes on the three major energy systems.

Heating and Cooling Properties of Medicines

Heating and cooling properties of medicines are very important because of their effect on the body during healing. Substances with heating effects dilate capillaries, causing increased circulation; substances with cooling effects constrict

67

capillaries, decreasing circulation. These effects are linked with the six tastes as follows:

1. Sweet, bitter or astringent-tasting medicines are cooling.
2. Sour, salty or pungent-tasting medicines are heating.

All exceptions to this generalization are in the Ayurvedic texts. If a sweet medicine has a heating as opposed to cooling effect, this will affect the medicine's activity.

In general, heating medicines strongly affect heart, brain and liver; cooling medicines strongly affect stomach, bladder and kidneys. By controlling the medicines' heating and cooling effects, a Vaidya can dilate or constrict capillaries in needed areas. In asthma, for example, the medicine dilates the capillaries in the bronchi; in menstrual cramping, the capillaries of the uterus are dilated to relax and soften muscles. Also, the Vaidya must be careful when administering heating medicines to a patient with an infection or metabolic energy overbalance because the condition could worsen. Cooling medicines given to a weak or emaciated patient can weaken him further.

Effects of Digestion on Medicines

Medicines often change during digestion which alters the effects predicted by taste. However, this phenomenon is limited to pungent- and bitter-tasting medicines. Some bitter medicines will, after a short time in the stomach, change to pungent and heat the body. Similarly, some pungent medicines will change to sweet. This effect can be very useful. For example, two normal effects of pungent medicines are to increase heat and cause slight constipation (metabolic energy overbalance). Ginger, which is pungent tasting, can be safely administered to patients with metabolic energy overbalance, even though they usually get only cooling medicines. The short heating effect will allow the other prescribed herbs to enter the blood quickly. After digestion, the ginger's pungency will become sweet and nutritive.

68

Specific Actions

Many medicines have specific actions unpredicted by their tastes, physical properties, heating and cooling effects or digestive changes. Such medicines are classified according to the results of empirical tests. The testing and discovery of medicines with specific actions has been going on for thousands of years. Some major specific actions, along with examples, are on the following chart:

Sanskrit	Specific Action	Example (Latin)
1. Dipanum	appetizing agent that doesn't aid digestion	*Piper chava*
2. Pachanum	a digestive agent which does not increase appetite	*Coriandrum sativum*
3. Dipana-Pachanum	a digestive/appetizing agent	*Plumbago zeylonica*
4. Samanum	an agent that restores balance to any of the three energies but will not cause overbalance	*Tinospora cordifolia*
5. Anulomanam	a laxative which cleanses the bowels and aids digestion	*Terminalia chebula*
6. Samsranum	a laxative which cleanses the bowels/ doesn't aid digestion	*Cassia fistula*
7. Bhedanum	a purgative	*Picrorhiza kurroa*
8. Rechanum	a purgative causing liquid stools	*Operculina terpenthum*
9. Vamanum	an emetic	*Randia dumetorium*

69

10. Sampodhanam	a purifying agent causing excretion of sour bile, gas and mucus	*Bauhinia tomentosa*
11. Chidanum	an expectorant	*Piper nigrum*
12. Lekhanum	an expectorant causing dryness	*Acorus calamus*
13. Grahi	a digestive/ appetizing agent which heats the body/tightens stools	*Cuminum cyminum*
14. Stambhanum	a coagulant	*Holarrhena anti-dysenterica*
15. Rosayanum	an agent that promotes immunity, quick cure, and rejuvenation	*Balsamodendron mukul*
16. Vajikaranum	an aphrodisiac	*Mucuna prurita*
17. Sukralam	an aphrodisiac increasing semen production	*Orchid incarnata*
18. Suksaman	an agent which permeates the finest tissues	*Piper nigrum*
19 Vyarayi	an intoxicating agent which first affects the body and then increases digestion	*Cannabis indica*
20. Vikasi	an agent that saps vitality	*Areca catechu*
21. Visam	a poison that increases the penetrating power of other agents	*Aconitum palmatum*
22. Balyum	a tonic increasing general energy	*Sida cordifolia*

23. Tridosaghna	an agent stimulating the brain to restore body balance	*Emblica officinalis*
24. Medhyam	a brain tonic which restores clear thinking and increases memory	*Conscora decussota*
25. Mutralum	a diuretic (for urination)	*Tribulus terrestris*
26. Krimighna	an anthelmintic (kills worms)	*Emblica ribes*
27. Vatagna	a carminative (expels gas)	*Ferula narthex*
28. Visagna	an anti-poison	*Santalum album*

Medicinal Use

Ayurvedic medicines can be divided into medicines to restore balance and medicines as agents for specific symptoms. Both types are used simultaneously if possible.

Specific medicines are used in accord with the results of empirical testing, while medicines following the rules of taste, physical properties, heating and cooling, and digestive changes are used to restore the three major energy systems. Specific medicines are symptomatic, while medicines which follow the pharmacological rules are general.

Examples of using general medicines are:

1. Any medicine sweet in taste, oily and heavy in property, and cooling to the capillaries will nourish the body tissues and circulation, energize the body and neutralize toxicity. It will help nutritive energy regulate nervous and metabolic energies. Such sweet medicines are healing and strengthening.

71

2.   Any medicine which is sour, oily and light to digest, and heating, regulates peristaltic movement, promotes digestion and stimulates the heart and other internal organs. It will help the metabolic and nutritive energies regulate nervous energy.

3.   Any medicine which is salty, oily and heavy to digest, and heating, increases appetite and digestion, dissolves blockages in internal ducts, and strengthens nerves. It helps nutritive and metabolic energies regulate nervous energy.

4.   Any medicine which is bitter, dry and light to digest, and cooling, increases appetite, helps regulate body temperature, purifies blood and helps nervous energy regulate nutritive and metabolic energies. Such medicines dry the body and stop pus formation and inflammation.

5.   Any medicine which is astringent, dry and heavy to digest, and cooling, promotes the healing of injured tissues, dries the body, tightens the stools and aids nervous energy in regulating nutritive and metabolic energies.

6.   Any medicine which is pungent, dry and easy to digest, and heating, increases appetite, controls abnormal growth, clears blockages of mucus and coagulated blood, and reduces allergic reactions. It aids metabolic and nervous energies in regulating nutritive energy.

Medicinal Plants

In Sanskrit, the basic Ayurvedic text on botany and medicinal plants is *Nighantu*. This text describes about 500 herbs, fruits and vegetables, detailing their identifying characteristics, their useful and useless parts, the seasons for collection, their tastes, medicinal actions and physical properties.

The plants used in Ayurvedic medicine grow in the five climates of India, Nepal and neighboring countries: alpine, sub-alpine, temperate, tropical and sub-tropical. They are classified as:

1. Fruit-bearing plants without flowers. Examples are: *ficus religiosa, ficus racemosa* and *ficus carica.*

2. Vines, creepers and climbers, such as *piper chava, piper longum* and *tinospora cordifolia.*

3. Fruit-bearing plants with flowers. Examples are *bauhinia variegata, cassia fistula* and *cinnamomum camphora.*

4. Plants which whither after going to seed, such as *swertia chirata* and *linum usitatissimum.*

Ayurvedic study of the botanical structure of the plants involves the properties of the root, bark, stem, wood, gum, juice, bud, flower, milk, fruit, ash, oil, thorn, leaf, shoot, tuber, rhizome, seed and terminal bud. Properties of these change with seasons, especially in the root, leaf, wood, tuber, bark, stem, fruit, flower and milk. For example, the medicinal value of the roots of large trees increases in summer; the medicinal value of their stems and new leaves increases in spring; the value of the bark, milk and tubers increases in autumn, and the medicinal value of wood, fruit and flowers increases in winter.

DR. MANA: "In 1955, when I finished my study, I figured out that my study of herbs had been limited to the Kathmandu Valley. I decided to do some herbal trekking and field work. My mother agreed to this idea and told me to go ahead. Also, she said that because I was an artist, I must paint the plants I discovered on the spot. So, for two years, 1956 and 1957, I went trekking. It took me two years because I had to paint and collect all of the different plants in their different seasons and locations."

"This experience actually changed my life and made me famous. Right after I came back to the valley with my collection of plants, I gave a big exhibition of paintings of medicinal plants. I invited the King to the exhibition, which was held right in our garden in the clinic. Thousands of people came to the exhibition and the King was very encouraging. He told me to continue my work and he gave me some royal awards. From this time my family began to reclaim its reputation which it lost after the death of our grandfather. More and more patients began to come to the clinic."

Use of Medicinal Plants

Plants are usually prescribed in powder form, decoction or by administering the juice of fresh leaves. Non-poisonous plants that are sweet, astringent, bitter or sour in taste can be used in quantities of 1-2 grams in powder form. To make a decoction, 15-20 grams of chopped plant are mixed usually with 5-10 ounces of water and boiled for 20 minutes.

Non-poisonous plants that are pungent are prescribed in powder form in quantities of 1/4 to 1/2 gram. For a decoction, use 1/2 to 1 ounce, and the same amount for juice of fresh leaves.

Poisonous plants are purified and prescribed differently. Examples are:

1. Aconite - steam in cow's milk or goat's milk for three hours. Dose: 10 mg.

2. Strychnos nux vomica - soak in vinegar for three days. Dose: 100 mg.

3. Cannabis indica - Dried leaves are fried in ghee (clarified butter) under moderate heat for 5-10 minutes. Dose: 200 mg.

Medicines made according to these rules are prescribed generally two or three times a day for internal use. It must be remembered that preparation of Ayurvedic medicines is difficult to master, requiring years of patient practice. The preparation of animal and mineral medicines is a separate discipline requiring additional training.

Summary
The sense of taste is the most important means to determine the medicines' effects on the three major energies of the body. Sweet-tasting medicines are nourishing; sour-tasting medicines are stimulating; salty-tasting medicines are dissolving; bitter-tasting medicines are purifying; pungent-tasting medicines are heating; astringent-tasting medicines are drying. Physical properties of medicines also are used to determine their effects on the body. Heavy medicines stimulate nutritive energy and light medicines stimulate nervous energy. Each of the six tastes is linked to the energy system it affects more powerfully and exceptions are noted.

Heating and cooling effects of medicines are significant, as are medicines with tastes and effects that change after digestion. Taste, physical properties, heating and cooling effects and changes after digestion help determine the medicines' general effects on the three energy systems. Medicines following these rules are classified as general medicines for balancing the three major energies. Medicines not following these rules are listed according to their specific actions and used to treat specific symptoms. If possible, general and specific medicines are both used in treatment. Plants are usually prescribed several times daily in powder form, decoction or juice of fresh leaves. Poisonous plants undergo specific purifying procedures before use.

Chapter Five

Diet and Hygiene

"The strength and lustre are enhanced of one who knows the proper diet and regimen for each season, and practices accordingly."

Punarvasu Atreya
Founding Ayurvedic Sage

The diet is extremely important in Ayurveda. In using the sense of taste, Vaidyas formed the basis for understanding how foods can be used to nourish, prevent disease and treat disease. Proper diet can help maintain balance among the three major energies. Ayurvedic study of diet includes: times for meals, food combinations, seasonal influences and so on.

Ayurveda presents a pattern for meals (See Figures 8 and 9) and within these models a great variety of meals can be planned that fulfill the Ayurvedic requirements for balanced nutrition.

These models, if used conscientiously, are the most important means of understanding how to provide balanced meals.

76

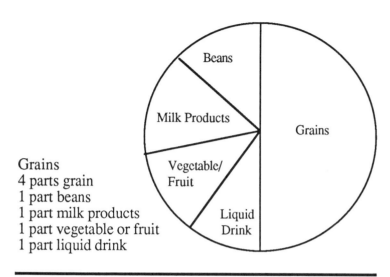

Figure 8. Model for a vegetarian meal

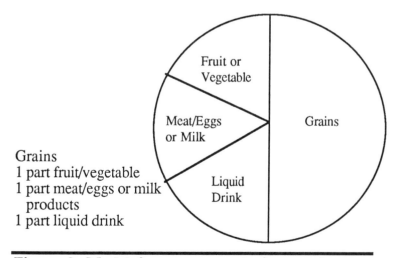

Figure 9. Model for a non-vegetarian meal

Balancing the Six Tastes

A second more subtle factor is balancing the six tastes. Each taste should be in each meal, if possible, or at least every day, and in certain proportions (see Figure 10) When tastes in a meal occur in such proportion, the meal is said to be regular and generally healthy. However, when one of the three major energy systems is overbalanced, altering the proportions of the six tastes will help restore the balance.

These guidelines shouldn't be interpreted literally. Rather, they are a model for balancing tastes -- especially spices. The amounts in grams and teaspoons are an idea of how much salt, bitter spices and pungent spices go into an average meal of 550 grams to balance the tastes. (Figure 10)

The Ayurvedic model differs from the usual Western way of eating in significant ways. The most obvious is the difference in proportions of the major foods. As in macrobiotics, about 50% of the food in a meal should be cooked whole grains such as rice, millet, buckwheat, corn, etc. The amount of salt should be less, and the amount of bitter spices more. Ayurvedic study shows that excess salt causes metabolic energy overbalance, which may partially account for the West's high rate of heart disease. Lack of purifying bitter spices accounts for many diseases, including unhealthy skin conditions. Excess tea and coffee, both bitter, may be a natural body craving to make up this deficiency, although the overuse of these drinks produces unhealthy effects.

Many Westerners eat almost exclusively sweet, sour and salty foods and such a diet overbalances nutritive energy and contributes to obesity, diabetes, sluggishness, etc., especially if exercise is lacking. An Ayurvedic diet attempts to balance tastes daily, although it is not necessary to add fresh spices to every meal, or include every taste in every meal.

Taste	Keyword	Weight	Percentage	Volume
Sweet	Nourishing	500 gr	90 %	_____
Sour	Stimulating	20 gr	4 %	_____
Salty	Dissolving	1 gr	1/3%	1/3 tsp.
Bitter	Purifying	1 gr	1/3%	1/3 tsp.
Pung.	Heating	1 gr	1/3%	1/3 tsp
Astrin.	Drying	27 gr	5 %	_____
		550 gr	100%	

Figure 10.   The regular diet

It's possible to see the effects of tastes by watching your body after eating specific foods or meals with a preponderance of certain tastes. After eating pungent (hot) spices, for example, you may notice a heating effect and an increased appetite. Garlic, for this reason, is a well-known appetizer. Drinking milk increases mucus exudation because it strongly stimulates the nutritive energy. After eating astringent foods, such as beans, there is a drying effect, while the slowed absorption in the mucus membranes of the intestines allows gas to form. The stimulating effect of sour foods, such as lemon or orange juice, also is apparent.

The person familiar with the six tastes can quickly restore balance to his body through diet. For instance, an increase in mucus production and sluggishness indicates nutritive energy overbalance. To counteract this, nervous energy must be stimulated and you must eliminate heavy, oily foods, milk products and excessively sweet foods, all stimulants of nutritive energy. Astringent, bitter and pungent foods and spices should be increased -- foods such as beans (astringent), honey (astringent) cayenne (hot), ginger (hot), and tumeric (bitter).

An extremely nervous and anxious person should increase sweet, sour and salty foods because nervous

An extremely nervous and anxious person should increase sweet, sour and salty foods because nervous energy, in this case, is overbalanced. And these foods counteract this con-dition by stimulating nutritive energy (as long as there are no other problems). Whole grains, cheeses, cooked veg-etables, and perhaps tomatoes can be eaten to nourish and calm. Cold and raw foods should be avoided for proper digestion.

According to the formula for major system balance {(Nervous energy <-> Nutritive energy)}-> (Metabolic energy), we can balance the body through diet as follows:

To Correct Increase These Tastes					
	sweet	sour	salty	bitter	pungent	astringent
Nervous overbalance	x	x	x			
Metabolic overbalance	x			x		x
Nutritive overbalance				x	x	x

FIGURE 11. Major energy systems and the six tastes.

Using Diet to Balance the Major Energies

The models are guidelines for preparing balanced meals. You should always have meals with balanced proportions of grains, vegetables, fruit etc. However, when one of the three major energy systems starts to overbalance, adjust the pro-portions of the six tastes. This is related specifically to the relationships between the six tastes and the three major energies. Guidelines are: to restore an overbalanced nervous energy, a heavier and more nourishing diet is required; to restore overbalanced nutritive energy, a drier and lighter diet is required, and to restore an overbalanced metabolic energy, a calming and purifying diet is required.

Diet for Nervous Energy Overbalance

Whenever nervous energy is overbalanced, use a heavier and more nourishing diet. Sweet and sour foods should be slightly increased and the salt intake should be doubled. Astringent foods and bitter spices should be used quite spar-ingly. The majority of foods should be chosen from this list:

1. Grains
   rice, wheat

2. Milk Products
   milk, butter, yogurt, cream

3. Meats
   pork, fish, chicken, duck, eggs

4. Vegetables
   onion, garlic, scallion, cauliflower, cabbage, tomato, spinach, lettuce, carrot, turnip, parsley, asparagus

5. Fruit (in season)
   lemon, mango, orange, pomegranate, lime, grapes, figs, guava, banana, coconut, apricot, pineapple, plum

6. Nuts
   walnut, cashew, peanut

7. Spices
   ginger, black pepper, cardamon, coriander, cinnamon, cumin, bay

8. Drinks
   water, alcohol (small amounts), tea, coffee, fruit juice

An example of a heavier and more nourishing diet is:
Breakfast
one egg
whole wheat cereal with butter and cinnamon
cooked fruit
tea

Lunch
tofu salad with onion, garlic, mayonnaise, lettuce, tomato
and parsley
cooked barley with peanut sauce
juice

Dinner
fish
brown rice with butter and soy sauce
asparagus
cooked spinach
wine

Diet for Nutritive Energy Overbalance

When nutritive energy is overbalanced, a drier and lighter diet is required. Bitter, pungent and astringent foods should be increased. Bitter spices should be doubled and astringent foods trebled. Sweet foods can be decreased about 10%, and extremely sweet foods and sugars stopped. Choose the majority of foods from this list:

1. Grains
   wheat, barley, corn, millet, oats

2. Beans
   mung, lentils, chick peas, soybeans, kidney beans

3. Meat
   eggs, wild game (little or no meat on this diet)

4. Vegetables
   leafy green vegetables, radish, eggplant, potato, garlic, asparagus, peas

5. Fruit (in season)
   apple, banana, guava, dates

6. Spices
   chili, ginger, black pepper, coriander, bay leaf, fenugreek, cumin, tumeric

7. Drink
   tea, coffee and hot drinks, water after meals

8. Honey should be included in all meals, about 1 tsp.

An example of a dry and light diet:
Breakfast
corn meal with cinnamon and dates
tea with 1 tsp. honey

Lunch
cooked beans with hot, bitter spices
lettuce salad with onion, garlic, etc.
cooked barley
tea with 1 tsp. honey

Dinner
corn and beans with spices
peas
vegetable soup
tea with 1 tsp. honey

Diet for Metabolic Energy Overbalance

When the metabolic energy is overbalanced, a calming and purifying diet is required, with increased sweet, bitter and

83

astringent foods. Bitter spices should be doubled and astringent foods increased about 50%. Choose the majority of foods from this list:

1. Grains
   rice, wheat, barley, millet, oats

2. Beans -- all types

3. Meat
   mutton, pheasant, eggs (little or no meat on this diet)

4. Vegetables
   mushroom, squash, cucumber, spinach, potato, lettuce, yam, turnip, carrot, asparagus, pumpkin, beet, cauliflower, cabbage

5. Fruit
   papaya, watermelon, pomegranate, banana, guava, pear, figs, grapes, coconuts, apples

6. Spices
   bay leaf, coriander, cumin, black pepper, ginger, cinnamon, cardamon

7. Drinks
   cold drinks, water, fruit juice

An example of a calming and purifying diet:
Breakfast
cooked wheat cereal with butter
cold fruit juice

Lunch
cooked beans with mild spices
brown rice with butter
cooked mushrooms
1 glass cold water

84

Dinner
cooked lamb (small portion)
yams
spinach and cucumber salad
cooked barley

Seasonal Influences

The seasonal weather fluctuations affect the balance between the three major energies. Nervous energy is aggravated by cold and humidity, metabolic energy is aggravated by summer (heat) and autumn, and nutritive energy is aggravated by cold (winter) and spring. Ayurveda says the increase in colds, coughs, etc. after seasonal weather shifts are caused by the failure to adjust to these changes.

Ayurveda divides the year into two-month sections to explain seasonal influences. However, depending on the geographical location, times and strengths of seasons vary. Use your judgment in interpreting the weather's effects on health. For example, the dietary adjustments suggested for winter (October-January) can be applied any time or place where the weather is very cold. Dietary rules for the rainy season, non-existent in the European and North American West, can be applied when it is raining or humidity is high. In tropical climates the heat in summer and autumn is very strong and in alpine climates the heat in the same two seasons is mild, but winter and autumn are very cold. All this must be considered.

In October and November, colder weather causes blood circulation to move to the inner parts of the body, away from the extremities and this creates extra heat in the abdominal area. Metabolic energy is increased and strengthened along with appetite. A heavier and more nourishing diet is required to stabilize the body, otherwise, the lowered blood circulation in the extremities can lead to joint pain, arthritis and other nervous energy problems.

People with strong metabolic energy usually have little difficulty with cold weather because their circulation keeps them supplied with heat. The nerve-natured people, or anyone with weak circulation, however, must be careful with their diet. The heavy and nourishing diet, with its increased milk products, meat and sour foods, creates mucus problems for some. The addition of honey, 1 tsp. per meal, averts this problem.

In December and January, cold weather is even stronger than in October and November and adequate heavy and nutritive foods must be eaten to avoid nervous energy disorders.

In February and March, the mucus accumulated in the body during the cold months is released into the ducts by the warmth of spring. Nutritive energy disorders, such as colds, asthma, loss of appetite, conjunctivitis, and sluggishness can result. A light and dry diet can counteract these.

In April and May, hot weather causes blood to flow toward the extremities and away from the abdominal region. This change can cause weakness, lowered appetite and digestive disorders, and can be corrected with a diet high in liquids. It also should include sweet, light, oily and cold food preparations, including ice cream. Sour, salty and pungent foods, meat, alcohol, and hot foods are discouraged because they can cause later metabolic energy disorders. A calming and purifying diet avoids these latter problems.

In the West, June and July are like April and May in the East in their effects. In the East, however, June and July is the rainy season and excess humidity causes the nervous energy and the digestive system to weaken. A heavy and nourishing diet can counteract this. Honey can help with the digestion of oily foods.

In August and September, bile and acids accumulate in the circulation, causing metabolic energy overbalance. In this season, a calming and purifying diet can be followed. Yo-od preparations and fish

ions and Diet

strong predisposition for
may forego the light and
ry and March. Similarly,
adopt a heavy and nour-
people should be careful
ess of the season.

	Nutritive	Diet
	----	heavy or regular
	----	heavy
	aggravated	dry or regular
	----	calming or regular
	----	calming or regular
	----	calming or regular
Humid	aggravated	----	----	heavy

FIGURE 12. The effects of the seasons on the three major energy systems

Antagonistic Foods

Certain foods, when eaten in combination, are antagonistic because they can cause sudden negative effects, or more

87

commonly, slow and progressive poisonous, overbalancing effects.

Ayurveda is cautious about using milk. Combining milk and fish, for example, causes heavy exudation and mucus formation. Milk can be beneficial, but because it will form a great deal of mucus, it should be taken by itself in small quantities or in cereals. Milk, in combination with other foods, can be very mucus forming. Adding cinnamon or ginger to heated milk before using will counteract this.

Ayurveda cautions against heating honey or using it in cooking, especially if it is from wild flowers. Heated honey will be absorbed without digestion and poisonous pollen gathered from certain plants may enter the bloodstream before the body neutralizes it.

Other prohibitions are taking hot and cold drinks together, which can cause colic, and eating burnt foods, which cause acidity. However, mild violations of these prohibitions are not usually harmful. Only constant violations create health problems.

Meals

Meals should be eaten regularly at fixed times during the day because this promotes good appetite and efficient digestion, and helps supply ample energy for work. Irregular meal times can cause indigestion, gas, acidity and nervous energy overbalance because the digestive system habituates itself easily. If you always have lunch at 12 noon, for example, the stomach tends to be empty each day at that time.

Too long a time between meals can create gas, and eating too frequently can mean indigestion or diarrhea. The small intestine and colon should not be empty, nor should they contain an inharmonious mixture of partially-digested and fully-digested foods.

Generally speaking, two full meals a day are sufficient for good health, but most people are accustomed to three or four meals. Nevertheless, major meals of the day should be about eight hours apart, with smaller meals or snacks spaced regularly in between.

The amount of foods eaten during meals depends on age, appetite, work habits, etc., but there are general rules. Meals including meat and/or heavy starches should end when the stomach is half full, while vegetarian or light meals should end when the stomach is three quarters full. People with active digestive power, such as hard laborers, may disregard these rules. During the winter, when digestive power is active even people with moderate digestion may disregard them.

Three Meals	Three Meals	Four Meals
small bkfst-8 am	full bkfst-8 am	small bkfst-7 am
full lunch-12 noon	small lunch-2 pm	full lunch-11 am
full dinner-7 pm	full dinner- 8 pm	snack-4 pm
		full dinner-8 pm

FIGURE 13.   Examples of proper meal schedules

Hygiene

Ayurveda emphasizes hygienic practices which promote physical and mental well-being. This emphasis is on cleanliness and avoiding excess. Neglecting such rules creates conditions which can lead to overbalance of the energy systems, while attention ensures health throughout your life. Hygiene and diet are necessary for successful medical treatment.

89

Hygienic Measures for Physical Health

The Ayurvedic texts are replete with practical hygienic measures. They list rules for cleaning the teeth (by crushing the stem of oleander or jasmine plants to make a brush), cleaning the tongue (using a scraper made of gold, silver or copper) and so forth. Sesame oil is recommended for a mouthwash once a day. Two or three drops also can be put in the ears at night to help the hearing.

Bathing is quite important, and should be followed by an oil massage or the application of oils, scents and perfumes. The feet, in particular, should be massaged with oil once a day. Sleep patterns should follow the natural cycle of sunrise and sunset.

Regular sexual intercourse is good for the body and mental well-being, but should be avoided during menstruation, on a full stomach, when tired, after hard labor, or in very hot or humid weather. A peaceful atmosphere is recommended.

Rules for Mental Health

In Ayurvedic thought, mental health is synonymous with virtue. The ancient texts made frequent and eloquent ref-erence to religious virtues, and similar lines of thought can be found in all texts up to the present. Honesty, courtesy, respect for others and truthfulness are the basic ingredients for mental well-being. Almost as important are numerous tracts which maintain that the sense organs should be trained and carefully used to avoid overstimulation or damage. Yogic methods of breath control, meditation, and cleansing all contribute to mental health.

Preventing Breast Cancer-An Example of Ayurvedic Hygiene

Ayurveda details very specific measures to prevent many diseases. An example of this is hygienic practices to prevent breast cancer.

1. Milking the breasts of newborn children
Immediately after the birth of any child, his or her breasts will be full of milk. This must be removed daily for a month, accomplished best by gently squeezing the milk out twice a day, morning and evening. This helps prevent blockages in the lymphatic ducts throughout life. And it is especially important for women, to prevent blockages at puberty.

2. Clearing blockages in the breasts
During menstruation, breasts often become enlarged and tender, later returning to their normal condition. If they do not, this indicates an abnormal condition from blockages in the blood vessels or lymph ducts. For the health of the breasts this condition should be corrected as soon as possible. Ayurvedic Vaidyas usually use a hot water bottle or roasted salt wrapped in thick cloth as a hot compress. An alternate method is steam bathing. During the treatment, sleeping during the day, interrupted sleep patterns and breast manipulation are prohibited.

3. Proper breast feeding
Ayurveda states unequivocally that breast feeding is essential to the health of the breasts. If a woman avoids breast feeding, it can cause blockage in the lymph duct systems and/or weakened nerve functioning. Both conditions contribute to breast cancer.

After childbirth, the mother can do a simple test of the purity of her breast milk. Pure milk dropped in water will dissolve. If it does not, this indicates milk impurities which may block or infect the mother's breasts. This can lead to disease in the child. To purify milk, use these herbs internally:

a. *cyperus rotundus* (nut grass)
b. *holarrhena anti-dysenterica*
c. *swertia chirata*
d. *tinospora cordifolia*

One teaspoon of tumeric cooked with each meal also will purify breast milk.

In case of stillbirth, premature death or if the child can't suckle, milk must be manually squeezed out for a few days. The practice can stop when the breasts are no longer stimulated. In general, breast feeding should be stopped when the child starts to have teeth.

4. Menstruation

Uterine and breast functions are interrelated and regular menstruation indicates healthy breast function. Menorrhagia (excessive menstruation) indicates metabolic energy overbalance and must be treated with one of the following blood purification medicines:

a. The powder of *Saraca indica,* 2-3 grams each time, or decoction of 3-4 ounces, taken three times a day.

b. Root of *Asparagus racemosus* (wild asparagus), powder, 2-3 grams twice a day.

c. The standard Ayurvedic compound chandraprabha is given twice a day with water, 2-3 grams each time.

d. 25 mg. of purified antimony and 2 grams of *Adhatoda vasica* taken with cold water 3-4 times a day.

5. Healthy circulation

Acidity, abnormal thermogenic functioning and excessive blood volume are three of the most common pathogenic conditions of the blood circulation when metabolic energy is overbalanced. Ayurvedic blood purification removes the acids, equalizes the circulation and heat distribution and restores proper blood volume. Laxatives, fasting and the diet for metabolic energy overbalance (See Page 83) are beneficial, as are the herbs *Santalum album* (white sandalwood) and *Balsamodendron mukul*. It is important to avoid all the practices listed on Page 56 which cause metabolic energy overbalance.

6. Sexual activity

The genitals and breasts have an obvious interrelationship. At puberty, for example, both breasts and sexual organs mature. Overindulgence in sex weakens the nervous energy, and, in particular, the chest nerves. This can cause distention, blockage and malfunction.

Summary

The general pattern for meals is the most important factor for a healthy diet and a second is balancing the six tastes. With practice, anyone can learn to balance his diet by using the sense of taste and correlating this with observed reactions in the three major energy systems. If nervous energy begins to overbalance, a heavier and more nourishing diet is required. If metabolic energy begins to overbalance, a calming and purifying diet is required. If nutritive energy begins to overbalance, a drier and lighter diet is required.

Weather also affects the body, and this can be managed with diet. Metabolic energy tends to be aggravated in summer and autumn; nutritive energy tends to be aggravated in winter and spring; and nervous energy tends to be aggravated in winter and by humidity. With this in mind, the year is divided into two-month segments with dietary recommendations for each. You must know your physical constitution to properly use these dietary rules. Antagonistic food combinations should be avoided and meals should be regular.

Cleanliness is necessary to good physical health. Regular bathing oil massage and proper sexual activity are very important. Honesty, courtesy, respect for others, truthfulness, courage and compassion promote mental health, as well as meditation, breath control, and cleansing and care of the sense organs.

Specific hygienic measures are prescribed by Ayurveda to avoid specific diseases. Milking the breasts of newborn babies, keeping the breasts free of blockages, proper breast feeding, regular menstruation and blood purification are recommended to prevent breast cancer.

Chapter Six

Treatment

"All the efforts of the physician, the medicines, the attendants and the patient, according to their qualities or abilities, for the restoration of equilibrium in the body tissues in the event of disequilibrium - this is the meaning of treatment. Profound medical knowledge, extensive practical experience, dexterity and purity - these are the four qualities of a physician. Power, suitability, comprehensive action and potency - these are the four qualities of medicine. Knowledge of nursing, dexterity, loving affection and purity - these are the four qualities of the attendant. Good memory, obedience, lack of fear and clear communication - these are the four qualities of the patient."

Punarvasu Atreya
Founding Ayurvedic Sage

Ayurvedic treatment is divided into two parts -- general treatment for the three energy systems and specific treatment for symptoms. In practice, both treatments are combined by prescribing various herbal therapies, either simultaneously or sequentially. For example, in an illness, a nerve tonic and a heavy diet may be needed to restore balance to the nervous energy, a laxative to stimulate elimination and a specific medicine to strengthen the liver. After five days, the laxative may be eliminated, a diuretic and a course of oil massage added, and the diet altered.

The skillful management of simple therapies in complex ways is guided always by the twin purposes of restoring balance to the three major energy systems (general treatment) and subduing symptoms (specific treatment).

General Treatment

The three major energy systems can be restored to balance by treating the correct energy in any overbalance. The formula for balancing the energies is:

{(Nervous energy <-> Nutritive energy)} -> (Metabolic energy). This can be broken down as:

1. Nervous energy regulates nutritive energy
2. Nutritive energy regulates nervous energy
3. Metabolic energy regulates combined nervous-nutritive energies
4. Combined nervous-nutritive energies regulate metabolic energy

In No. 1 above, if nutritive energy is overbalanced, it means nervous energy failed to regulate it. To restore balance to the nutritive energy, Ayurveda states, nervous energy must be stimulated and nourished until it heals and regulates nutritive energy.

We must realize that all body parts are interrelated and interdependent. Thus, Ayurvedic general treatment does not focus on the ailing body part. Rather, it stimulates and nourishes those energy systems that normally regulate it and allows them to do the healing.

Stimulation and nourishment are accomplished with medicine, diet, cleansing procedures and all other treatments of value in this process. This table explains in greater detail how foods and medicines with different tastes correlate with general effects on the three main energy systems.

Taste	Nut. Energy	Meta. Energy	Nerv. Energy
Sweet	strong increase	restores balance	restores balance
Sour	strong increase	strong increase	restores balance
Salty	strong increase	strong increase	restores balance
Bitter	strong increase	restores balance	strong increase
Pungent	decrease	strong increase	increase
Astringent	strong decrease	restores balance	slight increase

FIGURE 14. The effects of tastes on the major energy systems

The principles of general treatment are:

1. When nervous energy is overbalanced, nutritive energy must be stimulated and nourished, by prescribing foods and medicines which are sweet, sour and salty.

2. When nutritive energy is overbalanced, nervous energy must be nourished and stimulated, by prescribing foods and medicines which are bitter, pungent and astringent.

3. When nervous and nutritive energies are overbalanced, metabolic energy must be nourished and stimulated by prescribing foods and medicines that are sour, salty and pungent.

4. When metabolic energy is overbalanced, nervous and nutritive energies must be nourished and stimulated by prescribing foods and medicines which are sweet, bitter and astringent.

In addition to foods and medicines, of course, a life regimen must be followed which avoids more stimulation to overbalanced systems. In complicated cases, involving two or more energy systems, greater skill and knowledge are necessary to balance the three energy systems.

97

For foods and medicines to work properly, the body must properly assimilate and carry them to the needed sites. Accumulated toxins in the body will impair this process. Toxin accumulation occurs when there is an overbalanced condition, causing slowed digestion, slowed excretion and so forth. To overcome this problem and speed healing, five supplemental medical procedures are used by Ayurveda:

1. Inducing vomiting with emetics
2. Purgation
3. Inducing nasal secretions with errhines
4. Oily enemas
5. Herbal enemas

If the initial administration of any of these fails to properly cleanse the body, the procedure is repeated, but only after two preparatory procedures are used. The body is softened with internal applications of oil or ghee (clarified butter), followed by inducing perspiration, usually by steam.

Such procedures are related to the type of overbalance. Toxins characteristic of nutritive energy overbalance, salty mucus, accumulate heavily in the stomach. Cleansing the stomach with emetics is used in this case. The acidity characteristic of metabolic energy overbalance accumulates heavily in the small intestine and cleansing it with laxative or purgative medicine is very beneficial. The putrefactive gases characteristic of nervous energy overbalance accumulate heavily in the large intestine and cleansing it with enemas is valuable.

Specific Treatment

Specific treatment subdues symptoms. It does not follow the rules of energy system balance or taste-determined remedies in general treatment. Instead, plants and medicines are used according to their active principles and unique effects. In thousands of years of empirical testing, Ayurveda has discovered countless remedies for specific conditions.

For example, the herb *Acacia catechu* is used for skin diseases and the herb *Solanum xanthocarpum* is used for coughs. These medicines are given always with general medicines which restore balance.

For example, in sciatica, which is classified as a nervous energy disease, the patient is given general treatment and diet to stimulate his nutritive energy. He also is given lobelia, a specific remedy for sciatica that acts on the sciatic nerve.

Ayurveda frowns on treating symptomatically, without treating the overbalanced condition of the three major energies. Although symptoms may disappear, the untreated overbalance can express itself as another disease. For example, if a hemorrhaging patient is given medicine which quickly stops the bleeding, but does not address the cause, a severe overbalance in the metabolic energy will occur. The untreated overbalance can express itself later as a tumor or other serious symptom. Although neglecting overbalanced conditions may not always prove serious, it can easily result in overstimulation, poisonous effects and partial or complete paralysis. For example, it is especially damaging to suppress the symptoms of stomach ulcer or bleeding piles by symptomatic drugs.

Applied Treatment
Our treatment of Ayurveda, to this point, has been almost entirely theoretical. It has been simplified and divided into parts for clarity. Ayurveda, however, cannot be fully understood without full reference to specific applications to specific diseases. In these final sections, we will describe the diagnosis and treatment for: breast cancer, arthritis and herpes. All information from the preceding chapters will be used in this process.

Breast Cancer -- Ayurvedic Cancer Theory
Ayurvedic texts since the *Charaka Samhita,* centuries ago, have presented many theories and treatments for cancer and

99

abnormal growths. Most Ayurvedic authorities agree that cancer begins in the epithelial tissue lining the mucus and serous membranes of the body. This tissue is called "rohini" in Sanskrit, or "tissue with the nature of growth". Rohini tissue includes membranes lining the blood vessels and lymphatic system ducts, and the innermost skin layers. The tissue increases its activity when nutritive energy is overbalanced.

Ayurveda lists two pre-conditions for the growth of most cancers. These are:

1. Structural weakness in the lymph ducts and blood vessels in the connective tissues surrounding the muscles.

2. Various blood toxicities
The most common cause of structural weaknesses is pressure from blockages caused by heavy mucus exudation and accumulation. This results from daily or excessive indulgence in foods or behaviors which overbalance the nutritive energy. In the same way, indulgence in foods or behaviors leading to metabolic energy overbalance creates blood impurities. Such impurities manifest symptomatically as stomatitis, offensive odors, boils and pimples, acidity, weakness, anger, hot sensations, disorders of menstruation, etc.

Ayurveda states:

1.   If the pre-conditions of structural weaknesses and blood toxicity are present, and

2.   if any physical condition creates abnormal blood vessels (e.g. distention or injury), and

3.   these vessels start to dehydrate, this can result in abnormal growth of the rohini membranes, the beginning of cancer.

The breasts contain numerous ducts, and the rohini tissues lining the ducts are quite active because of the breasts' natural sensitivity. For these reasons, according to Ayurveda, they are very receptive to cancer.

As in all cancers, the beginning growth is localized, round in shape and appears similar to swelling. The roots spread to neighboring tissues and organs and the growth is constant, sometimes with pain. Ulceration with secretion of blood or serum is very common and difficult to cure.

Some Classifications of Breast Cancers

Granthi	-- smaller cancerous growths
Arbuda	-- larger cancerous growths
Vataja Granthi	-- small bluish cyst-like growth
Vataja Arbuda	-- large bluish cyst-like growth
Pittaja Granthi	-- small yellowish or reddish tumor-like growth
Pittaja Arbuda	-- large yellowish or reddish tumor-like growth
Kaphaja Granthi	-- small hard tumor
Kaphaja Arbuda	-- large hard tumor
Medoja Granthi	-- small fatty tumor
Medoja Arbuda	-- large fatty tumor
Mamsaja Granthi	-- small tumor in muscular tissue
Mamsaja Arbuda	-- large tumor in muscular tissue
Siraja Granthi	-- small tumor in vessels
Siraja Arbuda	-- large tumor in vessels
Vranaja Granthi	-- small growth within an ulcer
Vranaja Arbuda	-- large growth within an ulcer
Visarpa Granthi	-- small chain-like glandular growth
Visarpa Arbuda	-- large chain-like glandular growth

General Ayurvedic Treatment of Cancer

The general Ayurvedic approach to cancer treatment is to use five medical procedures to neutralize the factors causing overbalance and remove any damage. These are:

1. Blood Purification.
The blood is healthy when metabolic energy is balanced. Unhealthy diet, mental states, physical practices, etc., can overbalance this energy system and toxify the blood. The

blood is healthy when free of toxins, able to carry a good supply of nutrients and maintain a proper volume and heat distribution. Ayurveda uses these ways of purifying the blood:

A.   Laxative medicine -- Laxatives clean the intestines, reduce the absorption of bile and acids from the intestines, and help restore thermogenic functioning (heat distribution). A mild laxative medicine called "Triphala" is prescribed often at intervals depending on the patient's stamina. Triphala contains the fruit of three herbs: *Terminalia chebula, Terminalia belerica* and *Emblica officianalis*. (See *Planetary Formulas*, Page 165)

B.   Fasting -- Fasting stimulates digestive power, decreases the activities of the mucus membrane, reduces abnormal exudation and helps restore normal heat distribution. Moderate fasting is prescribed, depending on the patient's stamina.

C.   Bloodletting -- Bloodletting from the veins in the cancer area is beneficial because it removes the accumulated toxic blood. The blood should be removed from the capillaries.

D.   Blood purification medicines -- The most important means of cleaning the blood is purification medicines which restore natural properties and directly or indirectly neutralize the overaccumulation of bile and acid. Sandalwood compound is often used; it contains specific bitter and astringent herbs which balance metabolic energy. Alternatively, the bitter-dilatory herb *Tinospora cordifolia* is prescribed.

Sandalwood Compound

1 part	*Amomum subulatum*	1 part	*Cyperus rotundus*
1 part	*Cuminum cyminum*	1 part	*Coriandrum sativum*
1 part	*Mesua ferea*	1 part	*Piper longum*
1 part	*Cinnamomum zeylanicum*	1 part	*Glycyrrhiza glabra*
1 part	*Andropogon muricatum*	1 part	*Santalum album*
1 part	*Piper nigrum*	2 part	*Pterocarpus santalinus*

2. Healing the internal injury to the rohini membranes.
Internal medicines for healing the internal injury to the rohini membranes play a major role in the general cancer treatment. Several herbal compounds are used, depending on the condition. They generally contain Guggulu (*Balsamodendron mukul*) and purified mercury.

3. Removing blockages.
In the general cancer treatment, it is important to remove blockages caused by mucus and fluid secretions of the abnormal new blood vessels. Steam bathing, fomentation (external application of warm cloth soaked in medicines), plasters and compresses are prescribed daily. The fomentations, plasters and compresses are made from many substances, including lead, salt, radish seed ash, conch shell ash, tumeric ash, the milk of the *Euphorbia nerifolia* cactus and the purified seeds of *Datura stramonium*.

4. Increasing physical stamina.
A general tonic is essential in cancer treatment. With nutritive and metabolic energies overbalanced, the patient has greatly lowered vitality. Tonics stimulate nervous energy and improve general stamina. The standard Ayurvedic compound Yogaraja Guggulu is often prescribed.

Yogaraja Guggulu

Carum roxburghianu	1 Part	*Brassica campestris*	1 Part
Cuminum cyminum	1	*Nigella sativa*	1
Holarrhena antidysenterica	1	*Piper aurantiacum*	1
Stephania hernandifolia	1	*Emblica ribesl*	1
Scindaprus officinalis	1	*Picrorhiza kurroa*	1
Aconitum heterophyllum	1	*Clerodendrum serratum*	1
Terminalia chebula	13	*Terminalia belerica*	13
Emblica officinalis	13	*Balsamodendron mukul*	60
Tin oxide (*vanga bhasma*)	8	*Piper chava*	1
Silver oxide (*raypya bhasma*)	8	*Piper longum* (roots)	1
Lead oxide (*naga bhasma*)	8	*Cyperus pertenuis*	1
Iron oxide (*lauha bhasma*)	8	*Piper longum*	1

Mica oxide (abhraka bhasma)	8	Plumbago zeylanica	1
Iron ore oxide(mandura bhasma)	8	Ferula narthex	1
Mercury sulphide (rasasindura)	8		

5. Surgery

Surgery to remove an abnormal growth has value as a quick cure, but it's very dangerous. After surgery, any remaining abnormal cells will quickly spread throughout the body in the blood.

Specific Treatment of Breast Cancer

In addition to the general cancer treatments given to all cancer patients, Ayurveda has specific treatments. We will cover four of the most common forms of breast cancer. The Western medical terms are used because they are close, if not identical, to the Ayurvedic terms. The four types of breast cancer are:

1. Straja Granthi (Scirrhus Cancer)
2. Vrana Granthi (Ulcerous Cancer)
3. Mamsaja Arbuda (Myoma)
4. Visapra Granthi (Adenocarcinoma)

Treatment of Scirrhus Cancer

The specific treatment goal for scirrhus cancer in the primary stage is the rapid control of distention in blood veins and lymphatic ducts. The standard Ayurvedic compound Nayayana Tailam is prescribed for external massage along with Yogaraja Guggulu compound for internal use. (See Yogaraja Guggulu on Page 103). These must be used at least one month.

Narayana Tailam (oil)

Convolvulus arvensus	10 pts	Sida cordifilia	10 pts
Aegle marmelos	10	Stereospermum suaveolens	10
Solanum indicum	10	Solanum xanthocarpum	10
Tribulus terrestries	10	Sida rhombifolia	10
Azadirachta indica	10	Oroxylon indicum	10
Boerhavia diffusa	10	Premna integrifolia	10

Asparagus racemosus	63	*Sesame Oil*	63
Cow's milk	246	*Saussurea lappa*	2
Amomum sublatum	2	*Santalum album*	2
Sida cordifolia	2	*Nardostachys jatamansi*	2
Mineral salt	2	*Convolvulus arbensis*	2
Acorus calamus	2	*Vanda roxburghii*	2
Pimpinella anisum	2	*Cedrus deodara*	2
Desmodium gangaticum	2	*Uraria lagopoids*	2
Eryotania coronaria	2		

If the growth reaches the secondary stage before the patient seeks help, it is treated by cleansing the affected area and dissolving the lump. Thus, hot compresses are used, made from roasted salt and the milk of the *Euphorbia neriifolia* cactus. The salt and milk are wrapped in a thick cloth and applied hot to the affected area. The lump should be rubbed frequently with the fingers, using moderate pressure. Kaisara guggulu (Three Fruits compound) is essential to prescribe for at least three months to drain the dissolved sub-stance without negative side effects. This compound contains:

Terminalia belerica	64	*Tinospora cordifolia*	4
Emblica officinalis	64	*Piper longum*	2
Tinospora cordifolia	64	*Piper nigrum*	2
Baliospermum montanum	1	*Emblica ribes*	2
Operculina turpenthum	1		

If the abnormal growth does not disappear following this treatment, it is considered to be in the advanced stage. In this case, the standard Ayurvedic compound Gunjadayam tailam (an oil preparation made with *Abrus precatorius* and other herbs) is beneficial for external massage. The standard compound Kanchanara Guggulu (*Bauhinia variegta-Balsmodendron mukul* compound), *Raudrarasa* (purified mercury compound), and *Abhayarista* (a compound with fermented *Terminalia chebula* fruit) are prescribed with a general tonic for a prolonged time.

It is considered in the chronic stage when abnormal growth is painless, ulcerated, affecting the muscles of the chest and forming additional growths. It can, however, be suspended for several years with proper diet and hygiene along with the use of *Raudrarasa* (purified mercury compound).

Treatment of Ulcerous Cancer

The first step in treating ulcerous cancer is cleansing the ulcer with a decoction made from the barks of the Bodhi tree (*Ficus religiosa*) and the Banyan tree (*Ficus bengalensis*). Gunjadayam tailam (an oil preparation made with *Abrus precatorius* and other herbs) is then applied externally to heal the ulcer and slow the growth. The Three Fruits compound (See Page 105) and Kanchanara Guggulu (*Bauhinia variegata-Balsamodendron mukul* compound) are prescribed for internal use for at least three months.

Treatment of Muscular Cancer

In the preliminary stage, muscular cancer (myoma) is treated in the same way as scirrhus cancer, with the addition of an external application of a plaster made with sodium bicarbonate, radish seed ash and conch shell ash. In the advanced stages, the disease is incurable.

Treatment of Glandular Cancer

The major goal in treating glandular cancer (adeno-carcinoma) is controlling the inflammation. In the primary stage, a plaster is made from the powdered barks of the trees:

Ficus religiosa   (Bodhi tree)
Ficus bengalensis (Banyan tree)
Ficus glomerata
Ficus infectoria
Calamus viminalis

This is very useful for controlling inflammation. A warm plaster made with dried radish or the fruit of *Terminalia chebula* is very effective for relieving pain.

106

Kanchanara Guggulu (*Bauhinia variegata-Balsamodendron mukul* compound) is prescribed along with the Three Fruits compound for at least three months to control the abnormal growth. In addition, Sandalwood compound (see Page 102) along with a laxative medicine is essential to balance the metabolic energy.

In the chronic stage, a plaster made with Baladi (*Sida cordiofolia* compound) is beneficial. However, the illness is considered incurable if there is fever, loss of appetite or atropy.

Diet and Prohibited Behavior
The diet for cancer is on Page 149. The following behaviors are prohibited:

1. Conditions leading to emotional upset or anger
2. Working near heat or in the sun
3. Sleeping during the day or after meals
4. Overeating
5. Excessive sex
6. Exposure to severe physical vibrations
7. Strenuous exercise
8. Constriction of the breast
9. Breast feeding
10. Sedentary lifestyle

Arthritis

DR. MANA: "Arthritis is a nervous energy disease. When the nerves become overactive, the synovial membranes become dry and inactive. In arthritis, people actually lose their synovial membrane function. So, the Ayurvedic approach is to regenerate the membrane."

The primary cause of arthritis is an overbalance of the nervous energy which affects the nerves in the joints. Ayurveda distinguishes three types of arthritis: arthritis of the hand; arthritis of the knee; and arthritis of the foot, ankle, hips or wrist. If untreated, joint tissues deteriorate, causing stiffness followed by decay of the articular cartilage and the tendons. Atrophy occurs in the final stages.

Causes of Arthritis

Nervous energy can become overbalanced from any of the causes listed on Page 32. Any of these contribute to the development of joint pain. There also are four specific situations directly causing joint pain, swelling and/or inflammation. These are:

1. Putrefactive gases in the large intestine
According to Ayurvedic theory, whenever nervous energy becomes overbalanced, the large intestine becomes overactive. It also can result from stomach and small intestinal weakness. This overactivity weakens the functioning of the mucus membranes, leading to the production of putrefactive gases. These gases further weaken and irritate the nerves lining the large intestine. Nerve impulses are then transmitted to the spinal cord, resulting in nerve pain in the lower spine, hips, knees, ankles and feet. If these putrefactive gases are not eliminated, the condition can eventually develop into arthritis.

2. Deficiency of ojas
"Ojas" is a Sanskrit term with no Western equivalent. It is defined as "the final product of all metabolic processes", and it is an amber fluid. Without it, nervous energy does not function properly. It can be depleted by dysfunction in the bone marrow or by sexual excess. Such deficiency leads to nervous energy weakness. If this is untreated, it can develop slowly into degenerative arthritis.

3. Blood toxicity
Improperly digested food or improper metabolism builds up toxic by-products in the blood. These are sometimes expelled into the joints, where they help produce putrefactive gases. These gases can cause rheumatoid arthritis. Rapid development of rheumatoid arthritis is particularly common in a patient who has had rheumatic fever because the temporary arthritis of rheumatic fever permanently weakens the nerves of the joints.

4. Disordered uric acid metabolism
Sometimes nervous energy overbalance leads to a disorder in uric acid metabolism. When uric acid crystals accumulate in the joints, attacks of joint pain, or gout, especially affect the hands and feet. (Again, the clinically observed similarity between the concept of "disordered uric acid" and the Ayurvedic "Vatarakta," or "acid blood caused by a nerve condition" allows substitution of the Western terminology.)

These basic causes of joint pain, swelling and inflammation are more common in people over age 50, people with fragile health (especially those of nerve nature) and people living in cold climates.

General Symptoms of Arthritis

The primary stage symptoms are mild joint pain with or without swelling. These will usually appear during the winter, on cold or cloudy days, and in people with fever or debilitation. In its chronic stage, connective tissues degenerate and a progressive stiffness and atrophy follow. Severe pain and the inability to move the affected joint appear at the final stage.

If joint pain is because of gout or rheumatoid arthritis, it will be severe, and swelling will always be present. After finger pressure on the swelling area, it will assume its original shape when the pressure is removed, unlike edema where the area stays depressed. Arthritis usually presents other symptoms such as: weakness, loss of appetite, loss of weight, constipation, depression and numbness. These symptoms may develop into severe problems.

Specific Symptoms of Arthritis

Arthritis of the knee develops slowly, usually with inflammation, severe pain and stiffness. If there is a hyper-acidic or toxic condition in the blood, the inflammation can easily infect the knee. If the blood condition is normal, only general arthritic symptoms will appear.

Arthritis of the hand affects the tendons and the ligaments, resulting in pain, contraction of the fingers, and inability to move joints.

In arthritis of the foot, ankle, hip or wrist, the affected joint will lose its flexibility and become crooked. Pain, stiffness, abnormal cartilage growth and difficulty in movement accompany this condition.

Treatment of Arthritis

Generally speaking, the theory of treating arthritis is based upon increasing the blood volume and stimulating nutritive energy. Increased blood volume will supply extra heat and retard the accumulation of putrefactive gases. Stimulating the nutritive energy will increase blood volume because it controls the absorption of nutrients for cell growth. Finally, stimulated nutritive energy will control overbalanced nervous energy and repair the nerve tissue weakened by putrefactive gases. Use the following methods:

1. Oil Massage
Overbalanced nervous energy dries synovial membranes and reduces synovial fluid. This, in turn, stiffens the blood capillaries and limits the supply of nutrients to the nerves and synovial membranes. Oil massage counteracts this condition two ways. Oil lubricates and relieves dryness in the joint. Secondly, the physical effect of massage creates heat, which

dilates the capillaries and stimulates nourishment of the synovial membranes by increasing fluid secretion. A gentle oil massage with warm hands is prescribed twice a day and the oil must be absorbed completely into the skin. The standard Ayurvedic oil preparation Narayana tailam (wild asparagus oil with 28 other herbs, formula on Page 120) is usually prescribed, although with contraction of the joint, an alternate oil, made from black lentils, is used. If there is swelling, massage must be extremely gentle to minimize pain and avoid additional swelling.

2. Warm Fomentation
A warm fomentation helps soften the muscle tissue and clear the lymphatic ducts, although this treatment is not necessary in the primary stage of arthritis. In chronic arthritis, as muscles become stiff and contracted, it is necessary to promote their proper functioning. Such treatment should be introduced only after the oil massage, and it entails soaking cloth compresses in warm meat soup (prepared from any meat cooked in butter and oil), and applying these locally. Alternately, a warm decoction made from the leaves of *Sida cordifolia* is used. Afterward, the joint must be repeatedly manipulated to gain full benefit from the therapy.

3. Nervous energy tonic
The beginning stages of arthritis are curable by the sole use of oil massage. Chronic arthritis, however, requires internal medicines. Ayurveda uses several medicines which stimulate the nutritive energy. They will be either sweet, sour or salty in taste and dilatory on the capillaries. Such medicines tonify the nervous energy and are known as nerve tonics. The standard Ayurvedic compound Yogaraja Guggulu is most often used, one gram two or three times a day, for at least three months.

4. Warm poultice
A poultice can be made by pouring steamed meat or milk rice into a cheesecloth without draining. This is an alternative to the warm fomentation which follows oil massage, and is

111

usually used in cases of foot, ankle, wrist or hip arthritis. As with the fomentation, it must be applied warm, never hot to avoid burning.

5. General tonic
General tonics are valuable for arthritis caused by deficiency of ojas. This deficiency is common in middle or old age, or in a condition of general debility. Substances that increase weight and general energy are used.

6. Carminatives
Carminatives are aromatic herbs and spices that relieve or expel gas from the stomach and intestines; and arthritis caused by overproduction of putrefactive gases must be treated with carminatives. The standard Ayurvedic compound Ajamodadi churnam can be effective. Normal carminative spices should be used liberally: asafoetida, black pepper, bay leaf, cardamon, cinnamon, cloves, coriander, ginger, mace, mint leaves and nutmeg.

Ajamodadi Churnam
(2-3 gms. powder with warm water, 2-3 times a day)

Carum roxburghianum	1 pt	*Emblica ribes*	1 pt
Cedrus deodara	1	*Plumbago zeylanica*	1
Piper longum	1	*Piper nigrum*	1
Pimpinella anisum	1	*Terminalia chebula*	5
Sentaloide	10	*Ginger*	10
Mineral salt	1		

Diet and Prohibited Behaviors
The diet for arthritis is on Page 148. The following behaviors are prohibited:

1. Immersion in cold water
2. Interrupted sleep patterns
3. Anxiety or worry
4. Overindulgence in sex

5. Strenuous activities
6. Traveling in vehicles with severe vibrations, or being near machinery with vibrations
7. Overeating
8. Irregular meals
9. Sleeping on cold surfaces or in the damp
10. Sleeping naked, in the open or in a draft

Herpes

Ayurveda classifies herpes as caused by a nutritive and metabolic energies overbalance. There are two types: fever blisters, which appear anywhere on the skin, especially around the mouth; and venereal herpes, characterized by blisters on the genitalia. Fever blister infection strongly affects saliva and lymph fluid near the infection site, whereas, venereal infection affects the blood. According to Ayurveda, both types can be transmitted without contact: fever blisters through the air, and venereal herpes through water.

Symptoms of Fever Blisters

Slight fever, irritability, loss of appetite and inflammation of the skin are the first symptoms of fever blisters. After one or two days, watery blisters appear with itching on the inflamed skin. These break quickly, causing a painful lesion which forms a yellowish crust. The infection will disappear usually in four to five days without treatment. However, it tends to return repeatedly. The recurring condition can cause frequent colds, chest weakness and depression.

Symptoms of Venereal Herpes

Slight skin inflammation and blisters on the genitalia are the major symptoms of venereal herpes. The patient feels uneasiness, itching of the affected area and feverishness. After a few days, the blisters disappear without treatment. As with fever blisters, the infections occur again. This infection can cause degeneration of the genitalia, impotency and depression.

The Cause of Recurrent Infections

Herpes infection is not considered harmful in the early stages; however, the overbalanced nutritive energy continues to cause improperly digested food to enter the blood. This causes overexudation from the capillaries which accumulates in and on the tissues. The properly balanced body can excrete the waste fluid via the lymphatic system. A weakened or burdened lymphatic system cannot excrete the waste fluids quickly enough, and mucus blockages develop in the lymphatic ducts. Anyone with a finely-tuned digestive system, regular exercise and a proper diet generally will have no problem eliminating the infectional medium. These people can contract the disease and rid it from their bodies. Often, it will not return after the initial attack. People with malfunctioning digestion, poor diet or who are in poor physical shape may have the disease live in their bodies for a long time.

The Primary Causes of Excess Exudation

Any cause on Page 60 for the overbalance of nutritive energy can cause poor digestion and overexudation. Using antagonistic foods is another common cause (See Page 87). Most common is excess or daily use of meat, fish, milk and milk products, chemicals (additives and antibiotics), sour foods, vinegar, alcoholic beverages, fermented vegetables and salt. It is clear from Ayurveda why Western people have great difficulty with this infection.

General Treatment

The first step in treating fever blisters and venereal herpes is an external medicine. For fever blisters, a compound is made from oyster shell ash; for venereal herpes, a paste is made from *Acacia catechu..* This agent neutralizes and absorbs the infection around the inflamed area. It is applied daily until the blisters or lesions disappear.

To eliminate possible recurring infection, excess tissue fluid and mucus should be eliminated from the body. For this, blood purification medicines such as Kaisara Guggulu are prescribed.

Kaisara Guggulu

Terminalia chebula	67 pts	Terminalia belerica	67 pts
Emblica officinalis	67	Tinospora cordifolia	68
Balsamodendron mukul	64	Piper longum	2
Piper nigrum	2	Zingiber officianalis	2
Emblica ribes	2	Baliospermum montanum	1
Operculina turpethum	1		

Another blood purification medicine is *Alarasayana*, a compound of purified sulphur and several alterative herbs. The medicine's primary effect is increased circulation in the alimentary system, which increases digestive power and stimulates the lymphatic system. It restores natural properties to the blood, neutralizes toxins and reduces exudation. The Ayurvedic medicine stimulates the lymph and immune systems, which eliminate the virus. This is a long process and the medicine is prescribed several times daily for at least two months. The herpes diet (See Page 155), along with eliminating the behaviors causing both nutritive and metabolic energy overbalances (See Pages 60, 61) completes treatment.

Ayurvedic surgeons believe surgical removal of blisters is an alternate treatment to eliminate recurrent infection. Because the blisters are close to nerves, the operation is delicate.

Summary
Ayurvedic treatment is divided into general treatment and specific treatment. General treatment restores balance to the three major energy systems according to the formula {(Nervous energy <-> Nutritive energy)} -> (Metabolic energy). Healthy energy systems are nourished and stimulated to control overbalanced ones with medicines prescribed according to Ayurvedic pharmacology. Supplementary cleansing procedures - emetics, purgatives, errhines (for removing nasal secretions), laxatives - rid the body of toxins and increase the medications' effectiveness. Specific treatment

uses medicines for their pharmacological effects. Both general and specific medicines are used, if possible.

Breast cancer is the result of nutritive and metabolic energies overbalance. It can occur if there is structural damage in breast vessels/ducts and blood toxicity. These preconditions allow rohini membranes to grow, the beginning of cancer. Ayurveda has specific treatments for four major forms of breast cancer: scirrhus cancer; ulcerous cancer; muscular cancer, and adenocarcinoma (glandular cancer). Besides specific treatment, the general treatment consists of: 1) blood purification; 2) healing rohini membranes; 3) removing abnormal new blood vessels; 4) strengthening general stamina, and as a last resort, 5) surgery. Diet and prohibitive behavior also are addressed.

Arthritis is classified as a nervous energy disease which swells joints and damages synovial membranes. The major causes are: 1) putrefactive gases; 2) deficiency of ojas; 3) blood toxicity, and 4) disordered uric acid metabolism. Specific medicines are prescribed according to the nature of the arthritis, along with general treatment. General treatment includes: 1) oil massage; 2) warm fomentations; 3) nervous energy tonic; 4) warm poultices; 5) general tonic, and 6) carminatives. Diet and prohibited behaviors are addressed.

Fever blisters and venereal herpes are infections invited by overbalanced nutritive and metabolic energies. The infection can recur, causing lesions. A healthy body with good digestion and proper diet usually eliminates the infections. But someone with accumulated tissue fluid and mucus will have a lymph system too weak to eliminate the infection. Excess daily use of meat, fish, milk and milk products, chemicals, sour foods and salt cause overexudation and foster accumulation. The first step is eliminating excess exudation. External compounds are used to dry blisters, and powerful blood purification medicine is prescribed for months to increase digestion, restore natural blood properties and eliminate excess exudation. Surgery to remove blisters is an alternative.

116

Appendix One

Ayurvedic Medicinal Plants

This section introduces a few of the more common Ayurvedic medicinal plants. These plants grow in the four climates of Nepal and have been used by Dr. Mana's family for 700 years. The identification and study of these plants is controversial because of widespread disruption of Ayurvedic medical practice in past centuries, difficulties in identifying plants according to Sanskrit descriptions, substitutions of similar-looking plants by practitioners throughout India, etc.

The famed Bapalal Vaidya spent more than 30 years traveling around India clarifying many problems and I spent two weeks in India listening to him describe the anomalies. For instance, there are at least four plants known as "Rasna," an important Ayurvedic nerve tonic. Nevertheless, at least 90% of the important Ayurvedic plants are agreed upon.

GUNJA

Latin: *Abrus precatorius*
English: Crab's Eye,
Rosary Pea, Indian Licorice
Crab's Eye is a tropical and
sub-tropical small climber
with a slender and woody
vine. The leaves are
alterate pinnate
and the flowers rose to
purple. The seeds are
glossy, scarlet, black at
the base and poisonous.
Roots: sweet-tasting.
Used as a tonic.
Leaves: sweet- tasting.
Used in mouth for
hoarseness.
Seeds: bitter-tasting,
poisonous,
pungent, emetic, tonic.
Used as an aphrodisiac
when purified.

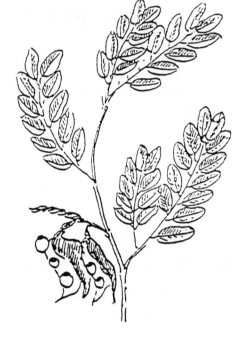

KHADIRA

Latin: *Acacia catechu*
English: Catechu Tree
The Catechu Tree is a
tropical and sub-tropical
small tree growing in
sandy areas and near rivers.
All parts of the tree are
bitter-astringent
tasting. It is used in skin
and urinary diseases and
throat problems. The
flowers are used in
hemorrhages.

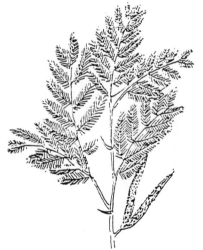

118

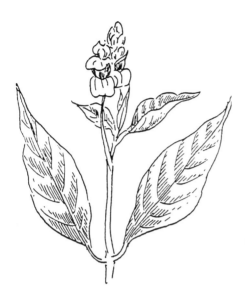

VASKA

Latin: *Adhatoda vasica*

Vasica is a perennial evergreen bush with lanceolate leaves, 8-10 cm, and white flowers. It grows everywhere, especially in temperate climates.

Leaves: bitter tasting, expectorant, diuretic, spasmotic. Used in hemorrhage, hemoptysis, hepatitis, fever, asthma,coughs and metabolic energy overbalance. One-fourth ounce of fresh leaf juice with ginger tea or honey is an excellent cough medicine.

Root, Flowers: bitter tasting. Used in abdominal tumor with inflammation.

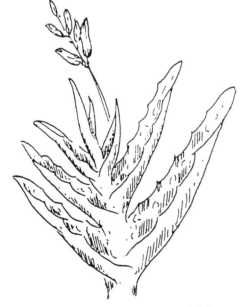

KUMARI

Latin: *Aloe barbadensis*

English: Aloe

This perennial is stemless and stoloniferous. The fleshy leaves are narrowly lanceolate, 1-2 feet long, with spiny teeth at edges

Leaves: bitter-tasting. Used as a purgative in liver and spleen problems and as an ointment for skin diseases or burns.

SURANA
Latin: *Amorphophallus campanulatus*
English: Telingo Potato
The Telingo Potato is an annual tuberous plant growing in shaded forest areas. The leaves are ovate to lanceolate, 30-40 cm long.
Tuber: pungent-tasting, stomachic, carminative and tonic. Used in hemorrhoids and tumors.

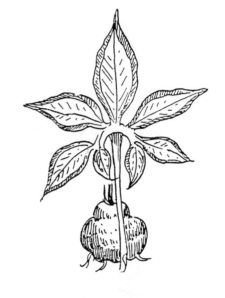

SHATAUARI
Latin: *Asparagus racemosus*
English: Wild Asparagus
Wild Asparagus is tropical and sub-tropical, thorny, perennial, and tuberous shrub, climbing to 20 feet.
Root: bitter-tasting, aphrodisiac, stomachic, tonic. Used in hemorrhage, menorrhagia, hermaturia, gout, inflammatory diseases of the heart and liver, and overbalanced metabolic and nervous energies' disorders. It is a brain tonic used in mental disease and epilepsy.

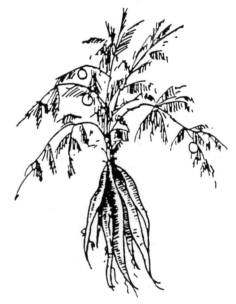

120

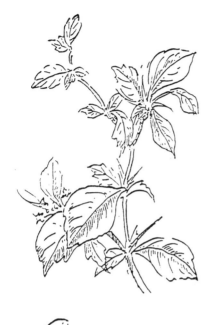

GUGGULU

Latin: *Balsamodendron mukul*

English: Indian Bedellium

Guggulu is a small tropical, thorny tree with aromatic gum. The flowers are red.

Gum: bitter-pungent tasting, diaphoretic, diuretic, demulcent, carminative, alterative. It is used in cancer, glandular swelling and nervous and nutritive energies overbalance.

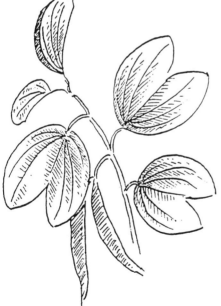

KANCHANARA

Latin: *Bauhinia tomentosa*

English: Mountain abony

The Mountain abony is a sub-tropical, medium-sized tree with emarginate leaves, 6-8 cm. long.

Bark: sweet-astringent tasting. Used in diarrhea, leprosy, glandular swelling and ulcer.

Seeds: tonic, aphrodisiac

KOVIDARA
Latin: *Bauhinia variegata*
Kovidara is a tropical and
sub-tropical
tree, with emarginate
leaves 8-10 cm. long.
Flowers: sweet-astringent
tasting. Used in diarrhea,
sprue and hemorrhage.
Bark: sweet-astringent
tasting. Used
as an emetic.

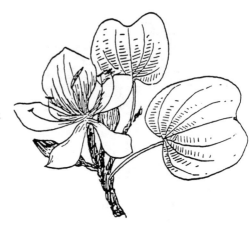

KUSMANDA
Latin: *Benincasa hispida*
English: Wax Gourd,
White Pumpkin
The Wax Gourd is an
annual creeper with a
long-running vine. The
leaves are broadly cordate-
ovate, angled and lobed
Fruit: sweet-bitter tasting,
nutritive, tonic and
diuretic. Used as a
refrigerant in
asthma, epilepsy and
hemorrhage. It has sedative
qualities.

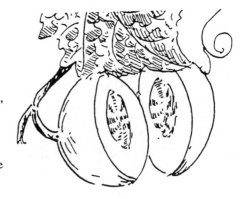

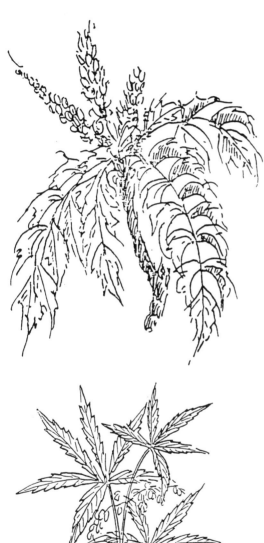

DARUHARIDRA
Latin: *Berberis nepalensis*
English: Barberry
Barberry is a perennial spiny shrub orsmall tree with yellow wood. The leaves are thorny and deciduous, and brightly colored in the fall. The flowers are yellow to red. It grows in temperate mountainous climates.
Bark: (condensed extract made from decoction of bark): bitter tasting. Used as a cleanser and anti-poison in eye,nose, mouth and ear diseases. Also used in menorrhagia, leucorrhea, urinary diseases and overbalanced nutritive energy. Used externally on sores.

BHANGA
Latin: *Cannabis indica*
English: Marijuana,
Hemp is an annual plant with a tough fibrous inner bark. The leaves have three to seven segments, and are narrowly lanceolate. All plant parts are bitter-pungent tasting. Used as a pain killer, anti-spasmotic and aphrodisiac. It helps in diarrhea and summer colds.

123

SWARNAPATRI
Latin: *Cassia auriculata*
English: Senna
Senna is an annual plant
with alterate pinnate leaves
which grows in tropical
climates in plains areas,
especially in
southern India.
Leaves: bitter-tasting.
Used as a laxative and in
metabolic
energy overbalance.

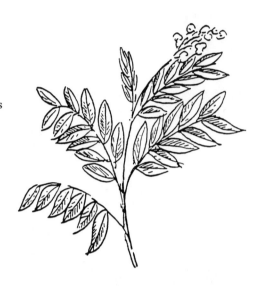

CHAKRAMARDA
Latin: *Cassia tora*
English: Sickle Pod
Sickle Pod is a perennial
bush which grows in
temperate climates. The
leaves are oblong-ovate to
ovate, 5-7 cm. long.
Seeds: pungent-tasting,
aperient, germicide. Used
in ringworm and skin
diseases.
Leaves: sour-tasting.
Used as plaster
for ringworm.

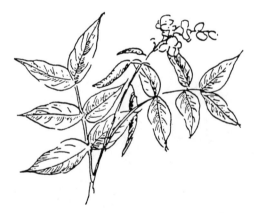

124

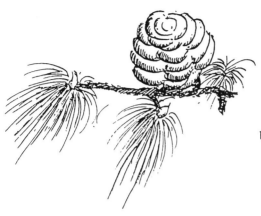

DEVADARU

Latin: *Cedrus deodara*
English: Deodar,
Himalayan Cedar
The Himalayan Cedar is
an alpine and
sub-alpine evergreen
with aromatic bark. It
grows to 150 feet with
branchlets drooping and
densely pubescent.
Bark: bitter-tasting,
astringent. Used in
fever, constipation and
nutritive and nervous
energies overbalance.

KARAPURA

Latin: *Cinnamomum
camphora*
English: Camphor
tree
A perennial evergreen
which grows to 100
feet. The branches are
yellow-brown, with
buds enclosed by
unbricate scales. The
leaves are alternate,
aromatic and ovate-
elliptic.
Leaves: (Crystalized
extract of leaves):
Used in mouth and
throat diseases. It
stimulates the
bladder and skin in
internal and external
uses.

MATULUNGA
Latin: *Citrus medica*
English: Citron
The Citron is a large thorny
perennial shrub or small tree
which grows to about
10 feet in mountainous sub-
tropical climates. The leaves
are oblong to eliptic-ovate
and the flowers are
clustered and purplish in
bud.
Fruit: two varieties, sweet
and sour. Used in chronic
diarrhea and alcoholism.
They are heart tonics and
appetizers.
Roots: bitter tasting. Used
in heart and uterine pain.

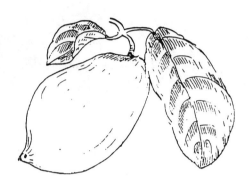

JIRAKAM
Latin: *Cuminum cyminum*
English: Cumin
Cumin is a tropical spicy
plant cultivated in plains
areas. The leaves have
thread-like divisions, and
the flowers are small - white
or rose.
Seeds: pungent-tasting.
Used as carminative and
digestive, and
for purifying the uterus.

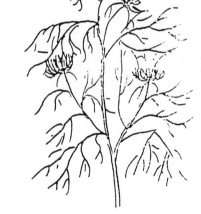

126

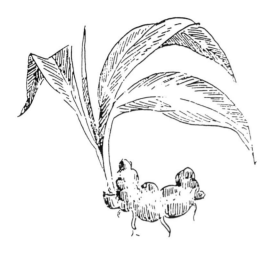

HARIDRA
Latin: *Curcuma longa*
English: Tumeric
Tumeric is a tuberous plant.
The rhizomes are short and
the tubers have yellow flesh.
The flowers are spiked to
7 inches with a terminal tuft
of white bracts.
Tuber: bitter-tasting.
Used as an anti-poison in
skin and urinary
diseases. Also used
externally for ulcers.
Tumeric paste mixed with
lime and saltpeter can be
applied hot to sprained,
bruised or inflamed joints.

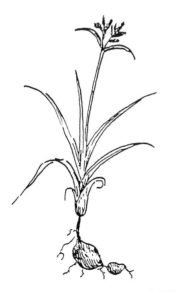

MUSTA
Latin: *Cyperus rotundus*
English: Nut Grass
Nut Grass is a tuberous
annual herb with fibrous
roots. It grows in tropical
climates. The leaves are
linear, 20-25 cm. long.
Tuber: bitter-astringent
tasting, stimulant, tonic,
demulcent, stomachic. Used
in diarrhea, enteritis, edema,
sprue, fever and metabolic
and nutritive energies
overbalance.

127

KRISNADHATTURA

Latin: *Datura metel,
Datura Stramonium*
English: Horn-of-
Plenty, Thornapple
The Horn-of-Plenty is a
glabrous annual herb with
ovate leaves, 10-15 cm.
long which grows to
about 5 feet.
Seeds: pungent-tasting,
narcotic, anti-spasmotic
and poisonous.
Purified seeds used in
rabies fever, asthma and
skin diseases.
Leaves: A paste from
leaves is used as
a plaster in glandular
swelling.

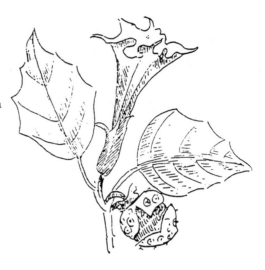

SUKSMAILA

Latin: *Elettaria
cardamomum*
English: Cardamon
Cardamon is a perennial
rhizomatous plant
cultivated in tropical
climates. The leaves are
20-40 cm. long.
Seeds: pungent-tasting,
aromatic. Used as a
carminative, mild
anti-poison and a
sedative. Also used in
body ache, cough
and vomiting.

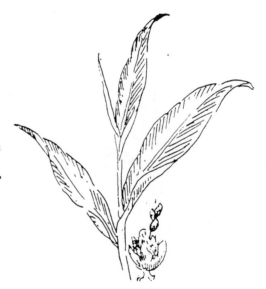

128

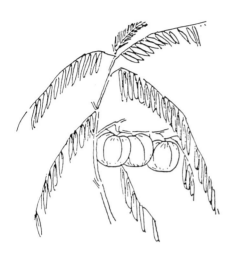

AMALKI
Latin: *Emblica officinalis*
English: Emblic Myrobalen
The Emblic Myrobalen is a deciduous tropical and subtropical tree which grows to about 50 feet. The leaves are linear-oblong, and the flowers small and yellow.
Fruit: sweet-sour and astringent-tasting, diuretic and laxative. Used in cough, asthma, throat problems, anemia, alcoholism, hemorrhage and fever. It is a tonic, especially for the heart, and an aphrodisiac and alterative. It is an ingredient of the internal cleaning formula Triphala.

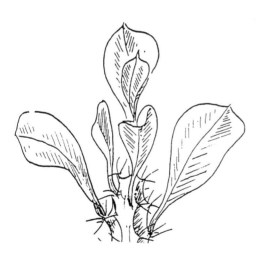

SNUHI
Latin: *Euphorbia nerifolia*
English: Milk Hedge
The Snuhi is a succulent cactus-like spiny tree. It is milky with a square stem, and has branches in whorls or slightly spiraled.
Milk: bitter-tasting, expectorant. Used as a purgative in abdominal diseases.

129

HINGU

Latin: *Ferula narthex*
English: Asaphoetida
Asaphoetida is a tropical perennial,
thorny plant with an aromatic gum-resin.
It grows abundantly in the desert of northern India
Gum-Resin: bitter-tasting, stimulant, anti-spasmotic, diuretic and aphrodisiac. Used as a carminative in gas and colic.

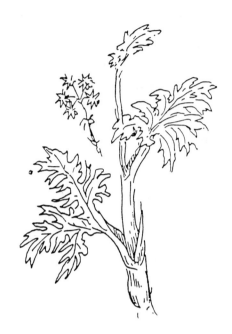

VATA

Latin: *Ficus bengalensis*
English: Banyan Tree
The Banyan Tree is a very large tropical and sub-tropical evergreen. The leaves are leathery, broadly ovate to elliptic, 10-15 cm. long.
Bark: astringent-tasting, tonic, cooling and diuretic. Used in diarrhea, bacillary dysentery, hemorrhage and as a plaster for bruises, sores and ulcers.

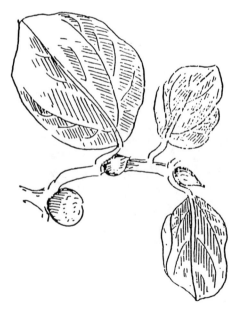

130

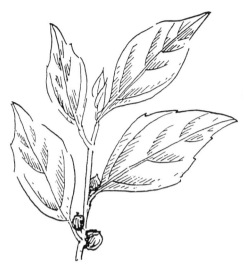

UDUMBARA
Latin: *Ficus racemosa*
The Udumbara is a tropical and sub-tropical perennial which grows to 60 feet. The base is rounded and the leaves elliptic to ovate-lanceolate.
Shoot: astringent-tasting. Used in diarrhea.
Bark: astringent-tasting, cooling. Used in urinary frequency, diarrhea, and as a plaster.

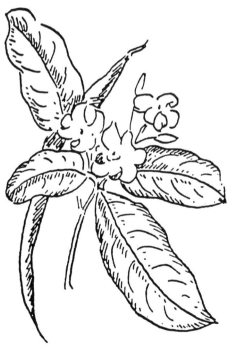

KUTAJA, IDRAYAVA
Latin: *Holarrhena anti-dysenterica*
English: Kurchi
The Kutaja is a small sub-tropical deciduous tree with leaves elliptic to ovate.
Seeds, Bark: bitter-tasting, stomachic, febrifuge and anti-thelmintic. Used in dysentery, fever, hemorrhoids, hemorrhage and diarrhea.

KATAKALAMBU
Latin: *Laginaria siceraria*
English: Bitter Bottle Gourd
The Bitter Bottle Gourd is a viscid pubescent tropical and sub-tropical annual creeper. The leaves are cordate-ovate, 15-20 cm. long.
Fruit: bitter-pungent tasting. Used as an emetic.

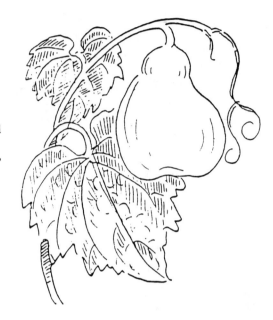

KAKANASIKA
Latin: *Leea aequata*
The Kakanasika is a temperate annual climbing shrub. It grows in temperate forests and the leaves are 6-8 cm. long.
All plant parts: sweet-tasting. Used as an alterative and tonic.

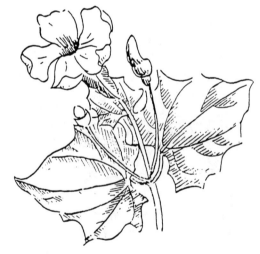

132

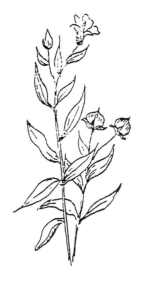

ATASI
Latin: *Linum usitatissimum*
English: Linseed
Linseed is an annual plant
cultivated in tropical areas.
It is known for its oil. The
lanceolate leaves are 2-3
cm. long.
Oil: sweet-sour tasting,
demulcent, expectorant,
diuretic and emollient. Used
in nervous energy disorders
for massage.
It is recommended for
cooking foods, urinary
diseases, or worms.

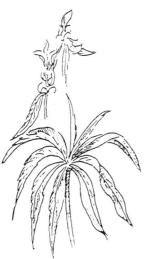

EKAVIRA
Latin: *Lobelia pyramidalis*
English: Lobelia
Lobelia is an annual tall
herb which grows in sub-
alpine forests. The leaves
are ovate-lanceolate and
alternate, and
the pink flowers have
bracted racemes.
All plant parts: pungent-
tasting. Used in sciatica and
back pain and in nervous
energy overbalance.

133

LAJJALU
Latin: *Mimosa pudica*
English: Sensitive plant
The Sensitive plant is a delicate tropical and sub-tropical plant with pink flowers.
All plant parts: bitter-astringent tasting, alternative and carminative. Used in diarrhea, hemorrhage and uterine dysfunction.

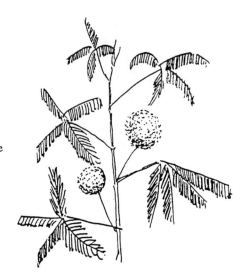

KAPIKACCHU
Latin: *Mucuna prurita*
English: Cowhage
Cowhage is a leguminous tropical and sub-tropical climber with poisonous hair on the pods. The leaves are alternate and lanceolate with large white flowers.
Seeds: sweet-tasting. Used as an aphrodisiac and tonic.

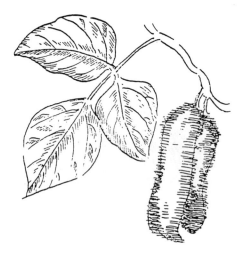

134

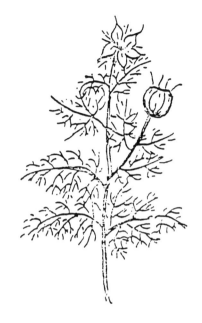

KRISHNAJIRAKAM
Latin: *Nigella sativa*
English: Black Cumin
Black Cumin is an annual
spicy plant cultivated
commercially. The seeds
are used for cumin spice.
Seeds: pungent-tasting,
aromatic, carminative and
appetizing. Used in
diarrhea, abdominal
colic and nervous energy
overbalance.

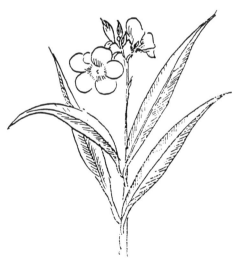

KARAVIRA
Latin: *Nerium indicum*
English: Oleander
The Oleander is an
evergreen erect shrub
with lanceolate leaves, 10-
15 cm. long. There are
many varieties depending
on the color of the showy
flowers, with terminal
branching cymes.
Root: bitter-tasting and
poisonous. Used
externally in leprosy.

135

SATAPUSPA
Latin: *Pimpinella anisum*
English: Anise
Anise is an annual aromatic plant with basal leaves, simple pinnate or alterately compound. The flowers are white.
Seeds: sweet-tasting, digestive, carminative. Used in colitis, fever and nervous and nutritive energies overbalance.

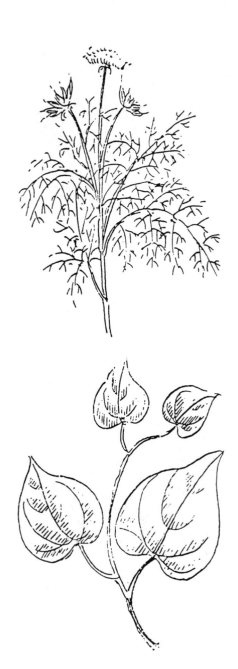

TAMBULUM
Latin: *Piper Betle*
English: Betel leaf
Betel is a tropical shrub vine, glabrous, with dioecious leaves, oblong-ovate to orbicular-ovate.
Leaves: bitter-pungent and astringent-tasting, aromatic, stimulant, and aphrodisiac. Used in painful menstruation. They can be chewed to clean the mouth after a meal.

136

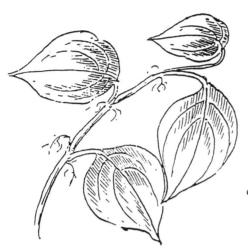

CHAVYAM
Latin: *Piper chava*

Chavyam is a sub-tropical creeper with a pungent odor which grows in the forest shade. The leaves are alternate-simple, and the flowers grow in cylindrical spikes. **Stems:** pungent-tasting, digestive and appetizing. Used in asthma, coughs, abdominal colic and nutritive energy overbalance.

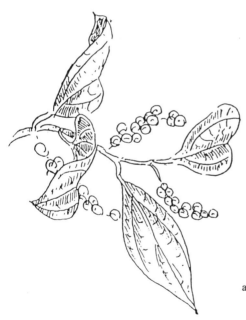

MARICHAM
Latin: *Piper nigrum*
English: Black Pepper

Black Pepper is a monoecious and dioecious climbing vine grown especially in southern India. The leaf blades are elliptic to orbicular-ovate. **Fruit:** pungent-tasting, digestive, carminative and appetizing. Used in coughs, asthma, worms, colic, and nervous and nutritive energies overbalance. It is combined with ginger root and Piper Longum to make the potent digestive and anti-mucoid formula, Trikatu.

137

AMLAVETASA
Latin: *Rheum emodi*
English: Himalayan
Rhubarb
Himalayan Rhubarb is an
annual with ovate-cordate
leaves, 20-30 cm. long,
and flowers greenish-
white or dark red. It
grows in alpine climates.
Rhizome, Stem: sour-
tasting, purgative.
Used in alcoholism,
neurasthenia, flatus,
asthma and to clean the
duct systems.
Fruit: sour-tasting.
Used as a heart
tonic.

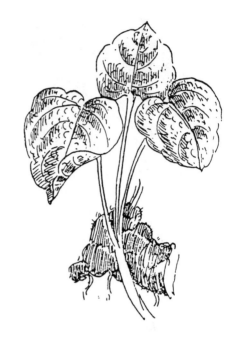

ROHITAKA
Latin: *Rhododendron
arboreum*
English:
Rhododendron
Rhododendron is an
alpine and sub-alpine
evergreen with oblong-
lanceolate leaves, 10-12
cm. long and red flowers.
Stem: pungent-tasting.
Used in enlargement of
liver and spleen.
Root: pungent-tasting.
Used in leucorrhea.

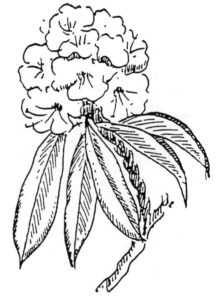

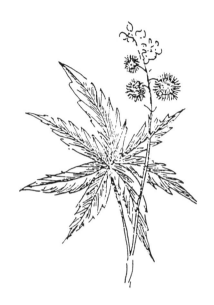

ERANDA
Latin: *Ricinus communis*
English: Castor Oil Plant
The Castor Oil Plant is an annual tall bushy plant with leaves 5-11 cm lobed. The flowers have no petals and many stamens.
Oily Seeds: sweet-tasting. Laxative.
Root: sweet-tasting, aphrodisiac and nervous energy tonic. Used in body ache and fever.
Plant ash alkali: For asthma and cough.

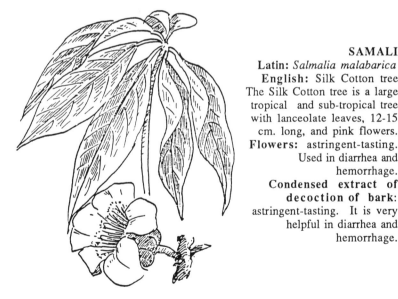

SAMALI
Latin: *Salmalia malabarica*
English: Silk Cotton tree
The Silk Cotton tree is a large tropical and sub-tropical tree with lanceolate leaves, 12-15 cm. long, and pink flowers.
Flowers: astringent-tasting. Used in diarrhea and hemorrhage.
Condensed extract of decoction of bark: astringent-tasting. It is very helpful in diarrhea and hemorrhage.

139

CHANDANAM
Latin: *Santalum album*
English: White
Sandalwood
White Sandalwood is a
tropical tree with
aromatic wood found
especially in southern
India. The leaves are
ovate to ovate-lanceolate,
8-10 cm. long. The
flowers are yellowish
turning to red.
Wood: bitter-tasting.
Used as a refrigerant and
anti-poison in
metabolic energy
overbalance.

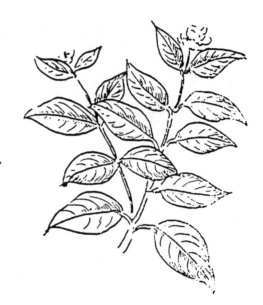

ASOKA
Latin: *Saraca indica*
English: Asoka
Asoka is an evergreen tree
found in tropical and sub-
tropical climates. The
leaflets are in three to six
pairs, oblong to oblong-
lanceolate. The flowers
are orange-red and fragrant
at night.
Bark: astringent, bitter-
tasting. It relaxes the
uterus and is used
in menorrhagia. It is also
used for metabolic energy
overbalance.
Flower: astringent-
tasting. Used in
diarrhea and bleeding.

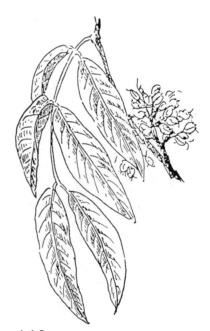

140

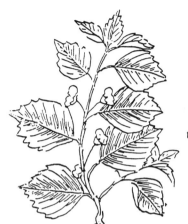

BALA
Latin: *Sida cordifolia*
English: Country Mallow
Bala is an annual small plant with simple serrate leaves and solitary yellow flowers in axillary clusters.
All plant parts: sweet-tasting. Used as a tonic in nervous energy overbalance. It is a valuable alterative for improving general well-being.

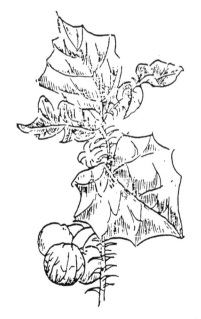

KANTAKARI
Latin: *Solanum xanthocarpum*
Kantakari is an annual thorny plant with leaves alternate, simple or compound, 10-12 cm. long.
All plant parts: sweet-tasting, aperient and alterative. Used in throat problems, coughs, cold, fever, chronic fever, body ache, edema and hiccough. It is a mild diuretic.
Fruit, Root: used in anemia.

141

KIRATATIKTAM

Latin: *Swerta chirata*
Kiratatiktam is an alpine and sub-alpine annual plant. It is glabrous with leaves opposite entire. The flowers are yellow.
All plant parts: bitter-tasting, tonic, stomachic and febrifuge. Used in fever and metabolic energy overbalance.

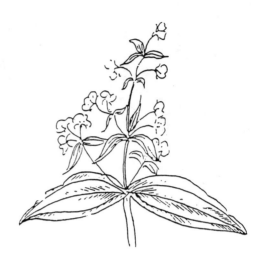

JAMBU

Latin: *Syzigium jambolanum*
Jambu is a middle-sized evergreen which grows in the hilly areas of temperate climates. The leaves are oblong-lanceolate, 8-10 cm. long.
Bark, Seed: astringent-tasting. Used in diarrhea, sprue, vomiting, urinary frequency, and diabetes.

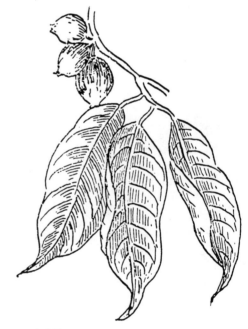

142

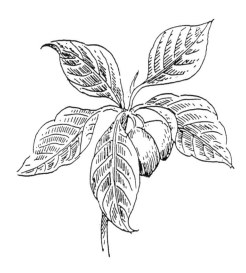

VIBHITAKI

Latin: *Terminalia belerica*
Vibhitaki is a large tree that grows in mountainous sub-tropical climates. The leaves are ovate-lanceolate, 20-25 cm. long.
Fruit: sour-astringent tasting, tonic, laxative. Used in cough, fever and nutritive and metabolic energies overbalance. It is an ingredient in Triphala.

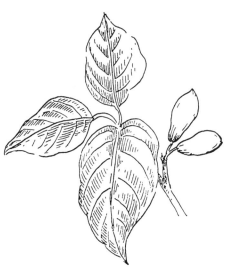

HARITAKI

Latin: *Terminalia chebula*
English: Myrobalan
Myrobalan is a sub-tropical tree with leaves elliptic to ovate. The flowers are bisexual and the fruit is a source of tannin.
Fruit: sweet-sour and astringent-tasting. Used as a laxative in fever, muscular defects, eye diseases and metabolic energy overbalance. Also used as an alterative for internal cleaning for good health in Triphala.

143

ASANA
Latin: *Terminalia Tomentosa*
Asana is a large tropical and sub-tropical tree with leaves nearly opposite, elliptic, and cuspidate, 5-7 cm. long. The flowers are dull yellow.
Wood: bitter-tasting, bactericidal, antiseptic, demulcent. Used as a blood purifier in skin diseases.

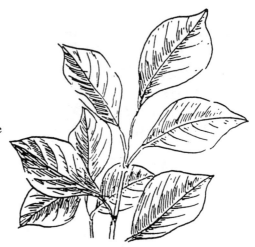

GUDUCHI
Latin: *Tinospora cordiofolia*
Guduchi is a long creeping vine found in temperate and sub-tropical climates. The leaves are ovate-auriculate, 15-20 cm. long.
Stem: bitter-tasting, alterative, diuretic. Used in urinary diseases, fever, toxemia, hepatitis and nutritive energy overbalance. It is an alterative for general good health.

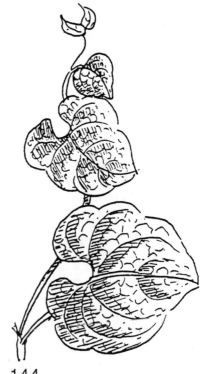

144

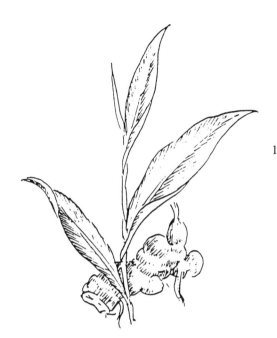

ARDRAKAM
Latin: *Zingiber officinale*
English: Ginger
Ginger is a cultivated spicy plant with yellow-green flowers, a tuber, and sheathing lanceolate leaves, 30-40 cm. long.
Tuber: pungent-tasting, carminative, digestive and aphrodisiac. Used in rheumatism, colds and allergies. It is an ingredient in Trikatu powder.

145

Appendix Two

Ayurvedic Dietary Prescriptions

These dietary prescriptions are used by Dr. Mana in treatments. Many are classical and others were developed by him or his family. They are to be used with a full Ayurvedic program. Foods are chosen with the same criteria as medicines. They are chosen for their effects on the three major energies and their specific effects. Food is an important factor in Ayurvedic treatment. For example, using heavy mucus-producing foods when reducing nutritive energy, or using acidic foods when reducing metabolic energy will neutralize or weaken the mild herbal medicines. Many of these prescriptions call for carminative spices (See Page 112). Food preparation is not covered, but an excellent manual is available from the Himalayan Institute. (See Appendix Three, Combined Therapy Clinic).

1. ABDOMINAL TUMOR:

Recommended Foods:
Rice, wheat/ mung bean soup with butter/ boiled green vegetables with oil/ radish soup with butter/ carminative spices/ garlic with all foods/ grapes, orange, lemon, tomato and other sweet-sour fruit/ milk products, including yogurt and whey/ alcohol in moderation after meals/ water with meals.

Prohibited Foods:
Fried or roasted foods/ meat/ beans/ corn, millet, oats/ hot spices/ dry foods such as biscuits/ tea, coffee or other hot drinks/ overripe fruit/ tuber roots.

Directions:
Fasting, irregular meal times and walking after meals are prohibited.

2. ACIDITY:

Recommended Foods:
Rice, wheat, barley/ bean soup, green pea soup/ boiled green vegetables/ papaya, orange, lemon, grapes, apple, watermelon, sweet plums, raisins and any sweet-sour fruit/ cucumber/ cashews/ milk, fruit juice/ water with meals.

Prohibited Foods:
Meat/ alcohol/ fried or roasted foods/ soybeans/ oily foods/ cauliflower, cabbage, radish/ vinegar/ biscuits or bread crust/ tea, coffee or other hot drinks/ candy, cookies or sweets/ chili/ oils/ organic acid foods such as pickles.

Directions:
Regular, fixed meal times.

3. ALCOHOLISM:

Recommended Foods:
Wheat, rice/ mutton, fish/ sweet-sour food preparations, including vegetables cooked with pepper, ginger or coriander/ green vegetables with butter/ sour fruit/ milk products/ fruit juices, small amounts of wine or beer after meals.

Prohibited Foods:
Sugar/ beef, pork/ chili/ millet/ beans/ tea, coffee or other hot drinks/ fried or roasted foods/ overripe fruit/ organic acids. Use salt moderately.

4. ALLERGIES:

Recommended Foods:
Rice, millet, corn, barley, oats/ boiled green vegetables/ ginger and black pepper with meals/ pomegranates, grapes, papaya/ tea and other hot drinks/ alcohol in moderation/ chili, garlic.

Prohibited Foods:
Meat, fish/ beans/ mango, citrus fruit, overripe fruit/ eggs/ cardamon/ coffee/ ice cream/ mushrooms, tomatoes, onions/ yogurt, cheese, cream/ organic acids, fermented foods, vinegar/ cold drinks or cold water.

5. ANEMIA:

Recommended Foods:
Rice, wheat, barley/ beans, lentils/ spinach, lettuce, beets, carrots, potatoes, green vegetables with carminative spices / butter/ meat soup with spices/ milk products/ grapes, raisins, figs, cantaloupe, pomegranate, cherries, banana/ water with meals.

Prohibited Foods:
Yogurt/ citrus fruits/ millet/ alcohol/ soybeans/ sesame oil/ vinegar/ tea, coffee and other hot drinks/ chili/ excess salt/ overripe fruit/ fermented foods/ fried or roasted foods.

Directions:
Regular, fixed meal times.

6. APPENDICITIS:

Recommended Foods:
Light diet with liquids/ barley, arrowroot flour and lentils with sugar or salt/ bread without crust/ boiled vegetable soup/ spinach, lettuce, asparagus, eggplant, fenugreek/ papaya, watermelon, grapes, cantaloupe/ milk/ warm water.

Prohibited Foods:
Citrus fruit/ oily foods/ butter, yogurt, cheese/ meat/ fried and roasted foods/ banana/ sweets, including jam, jelly/ vinegar/ alcohol/ hot drinks including tea and coffee/ chili, mushrooms.

7. ARTHRITIS:

Recommended foods:
Highly nutritive foods/ wheat, rice/ milk products/ meat/ oily and heavy foods/ sour fruit/ hot drinks, including tea and coffee/ alcohol in moderation after meals/ foods with carminative spices / dried fruit.

Prohibited Foods:
Leafy green vegetables, especially raw salads/ watery fruit such as papaya and watermelon/ pumpkin, yam, turnip, beets, potatoes, mushrooms, bamboo shoots, cauliflower, cabbage/ ice cream/ beans/ millet, corn/ mutton.

NOTE: Use rheumatism diet for rheumatoid arthritis.

8. ASTHMA
Recommended Foods:
Wheat, barley, rice (more than one year old)/ bean soup, chicken soup with hot spices/ potato, lettuce, parsley, fenugreek, watercress, asparagus/ tea, coffee and other hot drinks/ alcohol in moderation/ grapes, figs, dates, oranges/ honey with all meals/ water with meals
Prohibited Foods:
Milk, butter, yogurt, ice cream/ cold foods and drinks/ fish, pork, beef, mutton/ vinegar/ sour fruit/ squash, yam, mushrooms, pumpkin, cauliflower, cabbage/ all nuts/ coconuts/ all oily food preparations.

9. BLOOD TOXICITY:
Recommended Foods:
Rice, wheat, barley, millet, corn/ bean soup/ milk products except yogurt/ squash, pumpkin, asparagus, spinach, lettuce/ honey/ papaya, watermelon, cantaloupe, banana, grapes and other sweet fruit/ water with meals.
Prohibited Foods:
Pork, fish, beef, mutton/ alcohol/ salt/ sour fruit/ hot spices, including chili/ soybean products/ sesame products/ hot drinks, including tea and coffee/ potato, tuber roots, radishes, green vegetables (raw)/ yogurt/ vinegar/ oily, fried or roasted foods.
NOTE: Blood toxicity is in infections, toxemia, high blood pressure and metabolic energy overbalance.

10. BRONCHITIS:
See Asthma

11. CANCER:
Recommended Foods:
Rice, wheat, barley, corn/ mung beans, lentils, kidney beans, fresh peas, chick peas/ lettuce, spinach, watercress, carrots, squash, asparagus, fenugreek, artichoke, beet, cauliflower, cabbage/ milk products except yogurt/ papaya, cantaloupe,

grapes, cherries, figs, pomegranates and other sweet fruit/ cashews, almond, pistachios/ honey.

Prohibited Foods:
Beef, pork, mutton, fish/ bean pods, soybeans/ sesame seeds or oil/ tuber roots/ green leafy vegetables, potatoes, mushrooms/ vinegar/ sour fruit/ alcohol/ tea, coffee and other hot drinks/ overripe fruit/ salt/ fermented and acidic foods.

12. COLITIS:

Recommended Foods:
Rice (over one year old), wheat, barley, millet/ boiled green vegetables with carminative spices/ yogurt, cheese/ bean soup/ tea, coffee/ garlic, onion, scallions, parsley, anise, artichoke, asparagus/ pure drinking water/ pomegranates, raisins, figs.

Prohibited Foods:
Meat, eggs/ oily and cold food preparations/ milk/ alcohol/ vinegar/ sour fruit/ tuber roots/ fruit juices/ hot spices/ sugar, molasses, plums/ heavy foods.

13. CONSTIPATION:

Recommended Foods:
Rice/ bean soup with butter/ green vegetables, green peas/ all fruit except bananas/ milk products except yogurt and cheese/cold drinks.

Prohibited Foods:
Fried or roasted foods/ meat/ alcohol/ vinegar/ tea, coffee or other hot drinks/ hot spices/ yogurt, cheese/ bananas/ eggs/ millet, corn, wheat/ onion, garlic, scallion.

14. COUGH:

A. Dry Cough - Recommended Foods:
Rice, wheat/ meat soup with carminative spices/ beef/ well-cooked vegetables, potato/ fruit (only during daytime hours)/ tea, coffee and other hot drinks/ dried fruits/ milk/ boiled drinking water or warm salt water.

Prohibited Foods:
Raw salad, cauliflower, cabbage, radish, turnip, squash, mushroom/ peanuts/ coconut/ alcohol/ chili/ yogurt, cheese/ fruit late at night or early in the morning/ cold drinks.

B. Cough with mucus -- Recommended Foods:
Barley, wheat, corn, millet/ beans/ boiled green vegetables with hot spices/ potato/ chicken soup (fat removed)/ alcohol/ tea, coffee and other hot drinks/ ginger tea/ cheese/ honey.

Prohibited Foods:
Milk products, except cheese/ pork, beef, mutton, fish/ onion, turnip, cauliflower, cabbage, radish, beet, carrot/ sour fruit/ coconut/ peanuts/ raw salad/ oily food preparations/ cold drinks.

15. DIABETES:

Recommended Foods:
Wheat, barley, corn, millet/ well-cooked green vegetables with carminative spices / fresh peas, chick peas/ bean soup, chicken soup/ eggs/ milk/ fruit, dried fruits/ tea and coffee.

Prohibited Foods:
Sugar, molasses or sweets/ onions, mushrooms, potato, beet, tuber roots/ beef, pork, fish/ oats/ sesame oil/ animal fat/ yogurt, ice cream/ oily food preparations.

Directions:
Eat only small amounts of foods at each meal, with four to five meals per day.

16. DIARRHEA:

Recommended Foods:
Liquid diet/ lentil soup/ tomato, garlic, onion/ ginger, anise, parsley/ yogurt, cheese/ pomegranates, lemon, orange, apple, guava, persimmon/ tea and coffee (without milk)/ alcohol in moderation.

Prohibited Foods:
Heavy, oily foods/ meat/ green vegetables, raw salad/ watery fruit such as papaya/ milk products, ice cream/ cold drinks/ tubers, potatoes/ overripe fruit.

17. DUODENAL ULCER:
See Acidity

18. DYSENTERY
Recommended Foods:
Liquid diet/ barley, mung bean or lentil soup/ goat's milk, yogurt/ small amounts of bread or biscuits made with arrowroot flour/ spinach, watercress, asparagus, anise, parsley/ carminative spices/ pomegranates, figs, dates, small pieces of slightly unripe banana/ pure water.
Prohibited Foods:
Heavy, oily foods/ meat/ eggs/ milk products, except yogurt/ sour fruit, overripe fruit/ green vegetables, raw salad/ alcohol/ hot tea or coffee.

19. EDEMA:
Recommended Foods:
Barley, wheat/ lentils/ soybean products/ chicken soup with carminative spices / milk, butter/ dried radish soup, scallion, spinach, lettuce, asparagus, potato/ ginger/ tea, coffee and other hot drinks.
Prohibited Foods:
Fruit/ mutton, beef, fish/ green vegetables, raw salad/ salt/ yogurt/ sesame products/ sugar/ vinegar/ heavy or oily foods/ tuber roots, including beets and carrots/ squash/ cold drinks, alcohol.

20. EPILEPSY:
Recommended Foods:
Rice, wheat, barley/ vegetables cooked with oil or butter/ asparagus, spinach, lettuce/ milk products/ fruit/ eggs/ fruit juice/ sugar cane.
Prohibited Foods:
Meat, fish/ alcoholic drinks or other intoxicants/ beans/ hot drinks/ vinegar/ garlic, onion, scallion/ corn, millet, oats/ hot spices.

21. EYE DISORDERS:
See Epilepsy, no salt.

22. FEVER:
A. General Fever -- Recommended Foods:
Light liquid diet with barley and/or bean soup/ bread, arrowroot biscuits/ boiled vegetables, including spinach, lettuce, potatoes, asparagus, eggplant, bean pods, fenugreek/ papaya, watermelon, grapes, cantaloupe/ warm water/ warm milk/ tea, coffee and other hot drinks.
Prohibited Foods:
Sour fruit/ oily food preparations/ heavy foods/ rice/ meat/ fish/ yogurt, ice cream, cheese/ fried or roasted foods/ vinegar/ heavy sauces/ chili/ raw salad/ alcohol/ cold drinks.
B. Fever caused by injury -- Recommended Foods:
Heavy and nourishing diet/ rice, wheat/ meat soup/ milk products/ oil/ eggs/ boiled vegetables with carminative spices/ hot drinks/ dried fruit.
Prohibited Foods:
Beans/ soybeans/ corn, oats, millet, barley/ sour fruit/ cold drinks/ water fruit/ squash/ raw salad.

23. GALLBLADDER STONES, GASTRITIS:
See Acidity.

24. GONORRHEA:
Recommended Foods:
Liquid diet/ barley, rice/ bean soup/ boiled vegetables/ milk/ papaya, watermelon, muskmelon, cantaloupe, banana/ carrot, cucumber/ water (in large quantities)/ sweet fruit juices/ ice cream/ low salt intake.
Prohibited Foods:
Hot spices/ sour fruit/ meat, fish/ tea, coffee and other hot drinks/ vinegar, alcohol/ garlic, onion/ heavy sauces.

25. GOUT:
Recommended Foods
Rice, wheat, barley, corn, millet/ bean soup/ parsley, spinach, lettuce, asparagus/ potato/ boiled water/ milk/ boiled vegetables/ egg (one per day)/ banana, papaya, cantaloupe, watermelon.
Prohibited Foods:
Sour fruit/ meat/ fish/ green leafy vegetables/ alcohol/ fried or roasted foods/ soybeans/ vinegar/ fermented foods/ sweets/ pickles/ tea, coffee/ mushrooms.

26. HEART DISEASE:
Recommended Foods:
Rice, wheat, barley/ milk with water, butter in small amounts/ boiled green vegetables/ fruit, especially oranges, pomegranates, apples, mangoes and grapes/ fruit juice/ mung bean soup.
Prohibited Foods:
Hot drinks, incl. tea and coffee/ alcohol/ meat, fish/ roasted or fried foods/ vinegar/ oily food preparations/ molasses/ sesame oil/ hot spices/ soybeans/ tubers/ fermented foods.

27. HEMORRHAGE:
Recommended Foods:
Rice, millet/ mung beans, lentils, chick peas/ milk, goat's milk/ watery fruit/ raw eggs/ cold drinks, including fruit juice and sugar cane water.
Prohibited Foods:
Hot spices/ alcohol/ tea, coffee or hot drinks/ sour fruit/ vinegar/ salt/ meat/ fish/ green vegetables/ heavy, oily, fried foods.
Directions:
For the stomach and intestine, only a light liquid diet.

28. HEMORRHOIDS:
Recommended Foods:
Rice, wheat/ goat's milk, whey, cheese/ fruit/ dried radish soup/ onion, tomato, coriander, parsley/ cooked vegetables

with carminative spices / lentil soup/ water or cold drinks with meals.
Prohibited Foods:
Alcohol/ hot spices/ meat/ vinegar/ beans/ soybeans/ tea, coffee or other hot drinks/ fried or roasted foods/ oil.
Directions:
Regular, fixed meal times.

29. HEPATITIS:
Recommended Foods:
Rice, barley, wheat, corn, millet/ bean soup, dried radish soup, vegetable soup/ boiled eggs/ papaya, pumpkin, watermelon, banana, cantaloupe, grapes, figs and other sweet fruit/ sugar cane water or sweet fruit juice.
Prohibited Foods:
Oily foods or food preparations/ milk, butter, cheese, yogurt/ oil/ meat/ acidic fruit, such as lemon or orange/ alcohol/ coffee, tea or other hot drinks/ chili/ ice cream/ nuts.
Directions:
All food preparations must be boiled. If there is any nausea at the outset of the disease, lemons or oranges must be eaten for two or three days prior to meals.

30. HERPES
See Blood Toxicity

31. HIGH BLOOD PRESSURE, INFECTIONS:
See Blood Toxicity

32. HYPOGLYCEMIA:
See Low Blood Pressure

33. INFLUENZA:
See Fever (regular)

34. INSOMNIA:
Recommended Foods:
Rice, wheat/ milk products/ green vegetables/ fruit/ fruit juice/ bean soup with butter/ cold drinks.
Prohibited Foods:
Fish, meat/ hot spices/ tea, coffee and other hot drinks/ corn, millet, oats/ garlic/ vinegar.

35. KIDNEY DISEASE:
See Urinary Diseases

36. LEPROSY:
See Skin Diseases

37. LEUCORRHEA:
See Anemia

38. LOW BLOOD PRESSURE:
Recommended Foods:
Balanced meals of grains, beans and protein foods, along with spices (ginger, black pepper, cardamon, tumeric, bay leaf, cinnamon, nutmeg, etc.), vegetables etc.

39. MALARIA:
Recommended Foods:
Wheat, rice/ meat (especially beef)/ oily food preparations/ sour fruit/ vegetables/ highly nutritive foods.
Prohibited Foods:
Yogurt/ beans/astringent or drying foods/ alcohol/ excess salt/ vinegar/ fermented foods.

40. MENORRHAGIA:
See Hemorrhage

41. MENTAL DISEASES:
Recommended Foods:
Rice, wheat, barley/ mung bean or lentil soup with butter/ milk products/ fruit/ green vegetables, boiled or fried in butter/ cold drinks/ cold fruit juice.
Prohibited Foods:
Meat, fish/ alcohol, intoxicants/ hot tea, coffee or other hot drink/ vinegar/ oil/ garlic, onion or scallion/ hot spices/ corn, millet, oats/ peas/ soybeans.
Directions:
All food preparations must be extremely fresh and palatable.

42. MULTIPLE SCLEROSIS:
Recommended Foods:
Barley, millet, whole wheat bread/ beans/ cheese/ honey, honey water to drink/ bitter vegetables/ carminative spices/ food preparations with sodium bicarbonate or alkali of barley plant.
Prohibited foods:
Milk products in small quantities (avoid daily use)/ peanut butter/ sesame products/ meat, fish/ alcohol, vinegar/ liquid diet/ hot drinks/ starchy foods, especially white rice/ salt/ sweet or sour fruit.

43. NERVOUS SYSTEM DISEASES:
Recommended Foods:
Rice, wheat/ milk products/ meat/ oily foods/ sweet-sour fruit, dried fruit/ cashews, almonds/ hot drinks, including tea and coffee/ alcohol in moderation/ spices/ highly nutritive foods.
Prohibited Foods:
green vegetables, raw salads/ yam, turnip, cauliflower, cabbage, mushroom, carrot, potato/ watery fruit/ beans/ mutton/ ice cream/ cold drinks.

NOTE: Nervous system diseases include arthritis, neuralgia, neurasthenia, neck pain, sciatica, aphasia, etc.

157

44. OBESITY:
Recommended Foods:
Barley, oats, corn, millet/ green vegetables/ beans/ soybean products/ potatoes with hot spices/ sweet fruit/ spices/ water with honey in the morning and after meals/ tea or coffee
Prohibited Foods:
Rice/ meat, fish/ oily food preparations/ milk products/ sweets/ dried fruit/ alcohol.

45. PARALYSIS:
Recommended Foods:
Rice, wheat/ bean soup with butter/ milk/ boiled green vegetables/ fruit, especially sweet-sour fruit/ cold drinks, including fruit juice.
Prohibited Foods:
Hot drinks, including tea and coffee/ alcohol/ hot spices/ meat/ soybean products/ salt/ oil/ onion, garlic, scallion/ yogurt/ vinegar/ fried, roasted or heavy foods.

46. PEPTIC ULCER:
See Acidity

47. PNEUMONIA:
See Fever

48. PSORIASIS:
See Blood Toxicity. Also, filtered water, mung bean soup.

49. RHEUMATISM:
Recommended Foods:
Rice, wheat, corn, millet, oats, barley/ milk/ boiled green vegetables with ginger and carminative spices/ bean soup with ginger/ ginger tea/ coffee tea and other hot drinks.

Prohibited Foods:
Oily foods/ yogurt, butter, cream, cheese/ fruit/ meat/ alcohol/ pumpkin, turnip, yam, mushroom/ vinegar/ fried or roasted foods/ cashew, peanut.

50. SKIN DISEASES:
Recommended Foods:
Barley, millet, corn, wheat, rice (more than one year old)/ beans/ green vegetables with carminative spices/ banana, guava, apple, papaya/ tea, coffee and other hot drinks/ alcohol in moderation/ water after meals.
Prohibited Foods:
Milk products/ sour fruit/ fish, meat/ sugar/ sesame oil/ salt/ oily or heavy foods/ acid or fermented foods/ fried or roasted foods.
NOTE: Skin diseases include: ringworm, scabies, eczema.

51. SYPHILIS, TOXEMIA:
See Blood Toxicity.

52. TONSILLITIS, TYPHOID FEVER:
See Fever.

53. TUBERCULOSIS:
See Nervous System Diseases

54. URINARY DISEASES:
Recommended Foods:
Barley, corn, millet, wheat, old rice (more than one year)/ beans/ boiled vegetables with carminative spices/ cheese/ boiled eggs/ mustard oil, olive oil/ grapes, lemon, apple, banana and other fruit.
Prohibited Foods:
Alcohol/ tea, coffee and other hot drinks/ milk products/ oily, fried or roasted foods/ tubers/ sugar/ onion/ new rice/ well water/ meat/ fish/ nuts.

159

NOTE: Urinary diseases include albuminaturia, chylurea, phosphoria, etc.

55. WORMS:
Recommended Foods:
Wheat, corn, barley, millet/ beans/ boiled green vegetables with carminative spices and ginger, cucumber/ alcohol in moderation/ tea, coffee and other hot drinks (without milk and sugar)/ garlic, chili, black pepper, ginger/ papaya, banana, apple.

Prohibited Foods:
Sour or sweet-sour fruit/ meat/ fish/ milk products, except cheese/ sugar, molasses/ potato/ oily food preparations/ nuts/ ice cream/ excess liquids.

NOTE: Overeating is strictly prohibited.

Appendix Three

GRUNWALD & RADCLIFF PUBLISHERS is joining others in internationally exchanging information on Ayurveda. Please share the names, addresses and telephone numbers of groups and individuals involved in Ayurveda so we can incorporate them in our data base. The information can be sent to Grunwald & Radcliff Publishers at the address below:

Aside from scholars and scientists studying Ayurveda through anthropology and biochemistry, and doctors, medical students and allied health personnel eagerly learning more about Ayurveda, these groups are interested in promoting traditional Ayurvedic treatment:

AUROMERE
1291 Weber St.
Pomona, CA 91768
Auromere imports Vicco herbal toothpaste, Chandrika Ayurvedic Soap and many other Ayurvedic health care products and books.

AYURVEDIC ASSOCIATES
Alan K. Tillotson, M.A.
1008 Milltown Road
Wilmington, DE 19808, 302-994-0565
Ayurvedic Associates provides classes, seminars, workshops and home study courses on Ayurvedic medicine. Tillotson is the U.S. contact person for Vaidya Mana Bajra Bajracharya.

THE AYURVEDIC INSTITUTE
Vaidya Vasant Lad
Box 6265
Santa FE, NM 87502-6265, 505-982-5534
The Ayurvedic Institute offers extensive training programs in Ayurvedic medicine, as well as treatment under Dr. Lad, former medical director of the Ayurvedic Hospital in Poona,

India and author of **Ayurveda, The Science of Self-Healing.**

AYURVEDIC WELLNESS JOURNAL
141 Wyoming Blvd. NE
Albuquerque, NM 87123, 505-265-6432
The Ayurvedic Institute publishes the first U.S. **Ayurvedic Journal.** The subscription rate is $10 per year (four issues).

BAHAMAS AYURVEDIC REJUVENATION CENTER
3900 16th St. NW, Suite 507
Washington, DC 20111, 202-723-2372
Week-long and individually-tailored Ayurvedic treatment programs are offered by the center in a tranquil setting.

COMBINED THERAPY CLINIC
Dr. Rudolph Ballentine M.D.
Himalayan Institute - R.R. 1, Box 400
Honesdale, PA 18431, 717-253-5551
The Combined Therapy Clinic is directed by Dr. Rudolph Ballentine M.D. and Swami Rama. It provides Ayurvedic treatment with biofeedback, Western medicine, homeopathy and yoga. Dr. Ballentine's **Diet and Nutrition** has an excellent chapter on Ayurveda, and **Himalayan Mountain Cookery** by Martha Ballentine teaches traditional methods of food preparation, a key part of Ayurvedic dietary therapy.

EAST-WEST MASTER COURSE IN HERBOLOGY
Box 712, Dept. W
Santa Cruz, CA 95065
The East-West Master Course in Herbology, under Dr. Michael Tierra, N.D., C.A. is a masterful blend of Western, Chinese and Ayurvedic medical knowledge, covering all aspects of diagnosis and treatment. (For a sample lesson send $10 to this address). Highly recommended for the serious herbal practitioner. Dr. Tierra wrote **The Way of Herbs.**

162

Dr. Jeremy Geffen, MD
3256 Via Marin #17
La Jolla, Calif., 92037
Dr. Geffen is an author and student of Ayurvedic medicine and a student of Vaidya Mana Bajracharya.

GRUNWALD & RADCLIFF PUBLISHERS
5049 Admiral Wright Road, Suite 344
Virginia Beach, VA   23462, 804-490-1132
Publishers of Ayurvedic books, holistic health books and other New Age titles. Write or call for a catalog.

GURUDEV SIDDHAPEETH HEALTH CLINIC
Don Orlick R.Ph.
Ganeshuri, Maharashtra, India   401 206
21 Bhiwandi Exchange
A variety of Ayurvedic, holistic and allopathic treatments are offered at this beautiful ashram, only 20 miles from Bombay. The founder, Swami Muktananda, was trained in Ayurvedic medicine.

Jeffrey S. Hembree D.C.
Hembree Chiropractic Centre
328 Lynn Shores Drive
Virginia Beach, VA   23452, 804-498-8455
Hembree offers information on Ayurvedic diet.

Dr. Charles Lesley Ph.D.
Department of Anthropology
University of Delaware
Newark, DE   19711, 302-451-2000
Dr. Lesley is the foremost expert on the sociological and anthropological aspects of Ayurvedic medicine. He is the author of **Asian Medical Systems.**

163

THE MAHABOUDHA CLINIC
Vaidya Mana Bajra Bajracharya
Mahaboudha
Kathmandu, Nepal, Telephone 2-13960
This is Dr. Mana's clinic in Nepal. It offers free Ayurvedic consultation and the full range of Ayurvedic treatments. Patients are charged only for medicine. Inquiries, donations, etc. can be sent direct or through Ayurvedic Associates.

MAHARISHI VEDIC UNIVERSITY
14th St., NW
Washington, DC 20037 202-723-9111
This is one of the first Ayurvedic clinics and schools started by the Maharishi Ayurvedic Corporation of America.

WORLD MEDICAL ASSOCIATION FOR PERFECT HEALTH
Maharishi Ayurveda Corporation of America
107 S. Main St.
Fairfield, Iowa 52556, 515-472-8477, Telex 478304
MACA, under the direction of Maharishi Mahesh Yogi and Vaidya V.V. Dwivedi, is developing a large Ayurveda program worldwide. Plans include the opening of 50 Ayurvedic clinics in the United States. Information about their locations and services is available at the above phone number. Some centers are:

East Coast Center: 2112 F. St., NW, Washington, DC 20037; Midwest Center: 3201 Middle Glasgow Road, Fairfield, Iowa 52556; West Coast Center: 17308 Sunset Blvd., Pacific Palisades, CA 90272

MOUNT MADONNA CENTER
445 Summit Road
Watsonville, CA 95076, 408-847-0406, 772-7175
Regular Ayurveda training programs, clinics and workshops are held at the Mount Madonna Center.

PLANETARY FORMULAS
P.O. Box 533
Soquel, CA   95073, 408-438-1700
The Planetary Formulas Co. offers several potent Chinese and Ayurvedic herbal formulas, including some mentioned in this book. It has Triphala, Trikatu, Hinga Stahk and others. Its literature clearly explains how to use them properly. Call or write for a free catalog.

SANTA FE COLLEGE OF NATURAL MEDICINE
1590 Canyon Road
Santa Fe, NM   87501, 505-982-3038
Degree courses in Ayurvedic medicine, Oriental medicine and naturopathic medicines are given at one of the oldest schools of natural medicine in the United States.

If You Or Anyone You Know Has Been Treated by Dr. Mana in Nepal ...

Please write and tell us your story. Dr. Mana has treated thousands of Westerners in the past decade and we want to know what happened. Be very detailed and include medical records, if possible. Any material you want kept confidential should be so marked. The information will be used for an empirical record of successes and failures of Ayurvedic medicine for future publication.

Please send your name, address and phone number to:

AYURVEDIC ASSOCIATES
Alan K. Tillotson, M.A.
1008 Milltown Road
Wilmington, DE 19808
302-994-0565

Appendix Four

Healing Arts and Sciences Special ...

... An Ancient Spiritual Healing System for the New Age

Grunwald & Radcliff Publishers is developing and distributing a special section on Ayurveda, the world's third largest healing system. This section offers books, audio tapes, booklets and special courses for the novice and the master in Ayurveda.

The Handbook of Ayurvedic Medicine *Science of Life*
By Alan K. Tillotson M.A.
And Vaidya Mana Bajra Bajracharya
"It is the first book on Ayurvedic medicine that makes profound ancient truths of this system practically available and useful to Westerners." **Dr. Michael Tierra, C.A., N.D., Author, The Way of Herbs**

[The book is] " a fine introduction to this system of medicine .. providing a wealth of information that has previously not been readily accessible to people in English-speaking countries." **Dr. Robert M. Hall M.D., DE**

The Handbook of Ayurvedic Medicine *Science of Life* is a reference and study aid introducing an ancient healing system of Nepal and India which stresses diet/nutrition, mental discipline, hygiene, herbs and other natural medicines. This self-help, health book guides readers through Ayurveda, the world's third largest medical system (Western and Chinese medicines are larger), as seen through the work of Dr. Mana, a prominent practitioner in Nepal.

167

Ayurveda (meaning "science of life") stresses healing through maintaining the body's balance of nervous, circulatory and metabolic energy systems. Its research and beliefs are steeped in the rich understandings of Buddhist and Eastern philosophy linking body and mind to proper lifestyle and nutrition.

The Ayurvedic physician uses *"the rich and complex repertory of Ayurvedic medicine herbs and mineral drugs, in conjunction with specialized diet modification and various cleansing practices, to restore the various elements to their proper balance."* -- **Dr. Jeremy Geffen M.D., La Jolla, CA**

The author is a national consultant in and teacher about Ayurvedic medicine and lives in Wilmington, DE. He is a recognized authority in t'ai chi.

5 1/2 x 8 1/2 Softcover * 200 pages * $8.95 * ISBN 0-915133-08-3
Hardcover * 200 pages * $14.95 * ISBN 0-915133-09-1
Coming Soon...
Dr. Mana: Nepalese Ayurvedic Healer ---- By Alan K. Tillotson M.A. Trade Paper * $6.95 * ISBN 0-915133-07-5
Hardcover * $10.95 * ISBN 0-915133-17-2

- -

Ayurvedic Associates
Wilmington, DE, U.S.A.
offers: Dr. Mana's Ayurvedic Treatment (With Alan K. Tillotson, M.A.)
The Associates offers audio tapes and booklets on the Ayurvedic approach to diseases, in response to the interest of Dr. Mana's Western patients and to make the public more aware of Ayurveda. Each tape has a brief synopsis of Ayurvedic Herbal Theory, a simple description of Ayurvedic diagnosis, methods of prevention and the course of treatment, therapies, diet, etc. for each disease.

Tape Name	Price
Arthritis	7.95
Breast Cancer	7.95
Hepatitis/Jaundice	7.95
Diabetes	7.95
Herpes -- Oral/Genital	7.95
Hypertension	7.95
Leukoderma (Loss of Skin Pigmentation)	7.95
Hypoglycemia and Low Blood Pressure	7.95
Migraine Headaches	7.95
Multiple Sclerosis	7.95
Psoriasis	7.95
Asthma	7.95
Hay Fever	7.95
Hemorrhoids	7.95
Varicose Veins	7.95
Anemia	7.95

* Booklets available upon request, please send for price information.

For orders of 5 or more deduct a 25% discount $_____
Virginia residents add 6% sales tax $_____
Add $1.75 for postage/handling for first five items and
$.50 for more than five items $_____
Total Amount $_____
(Make check or money order payable to: Global Communications Associates, Inc.)

Please send order to: Global Communications Associates, Inc., 5049 Admiral Wright Road, Suite 344, Virginia Beach, VA 23462. Allow eight weeks for shipment.

Advanced Course in Ayurvedic Treatment of Serious Diseases
By Alan K.Tillotson and Vaidya Mana Bajra Bajracharya

The Advanced Course covers in detail the proven techniques used by Dr. Mana in Nepal. They are the result of the family's 700 years of medical practice which led the King of Nepal to appoint Dr. Mana's grandfather as the royal physician and King Birendra Bir Bikram Shah Dev, the current king, to choose Dr. Mana to head the Ayurveda section of the Royal Nepalese Academy of Science and Technology.

The first section of the curriculum presents in greater detail the materials in **The Handbook of Ayurvedic Medicine** *Science of Life*. Six lessons will cover: Ayurvedic analyses of 200 common foods (grains, fruits, nuts, drinks, vegetables); how to understand Vata, Pitta and Kapha in yourself and others; Ayurvedic teaching mythology; and Ayurvedic anatomy, physiology, hygiene and psychology.

The second section introduces the Ayurvedic medicines. Twelve lessons cover about 150 Ayurvedic medicinal plants, animals and birds, and minerals and gems used for treatment; common Ayurvedic medicines and how to use them; Ayurvedic home treatments, and medicine preparation.

The third section will provide detailed and practical treatises on the Ayurvedic treatments used by Dr. Mana for: herpes, hemorrhoids, hay fever and allergies, multiple sclerosis, breast cancer, psoriasis, diabetes, jaundice and hepatitis, anemia, leukoderma, migraine headaches, varicose veins, high blood pressure, low blood pressure, hypoglycemia, arthritis and asthma -- 16 lessons. Each lesson will cover the cause of the disease, its symptoms, prevention and the medicines used. Much of the information can be found nowhere else. Also included will be sections on using Chinese alternatives for each disease, written by Dr. Michael Tierra C.A., N.D., author of **The Way of Herbs.** The final lesson teaches the user of Ayurvedic diagnosis and theory about common Western herbs, such as the Dr. Christopher formulas and the Planetary Formulas.

The course may be paid for in three installments of $125 C.O.D. each or bought complete for $295 C.O.D. -- a 22% savings. This will include the lessons in booklet and tape form, charts and diagrams and supplementary materials. Fifty percent of the author's royalties go to the Mahaboudha Clinic to support its work. Please send orders to: Global Communications Associates, Inc., 5049 Admiral Wright Road, Suite 344, Virginia Beach, VA 23462.

References

1.   The Hindus use this name to designate themselves and other speakers of Indo-Iranian languages.

2.   P. Kutumbia, **Ancient Indian Medicine** (New Delhi: Orient Longman's Ltd., 1962) p. i.

3.   B. Dash, **Fundamentals of Ayurvedic Medicine** (Delhi, Bansal, 1978) p. 8.

4.   Kutumbia, p. xiii.

5.   Dr. Mana showed me this text in his library in June 1980.

6.   Kutumbia, p. 167.

7.   Kutumbia, p. 167.

8.   A modern anatomist would be quick to point out the errors which result from this ancient method. Dr. Mana spent a great deal of time studying modern anatomy, which he admires. At the same time, he thinks Ayurvedic doctors do not need to know everything modern science has. He told me that it is enough to know the major arteries, nerves, glands and organs, etc. Vaidyas do not need to "know the name of every capillary and blood cell."

9.   G. Murti, **The Science and Art of Indian Medicine,** (Adyar: Theosophical Press, 1948), p. 155.

10. Marc Edmund Jones, **Occult Philosophy,** (Baltimore, Md.: Schneidereith and Sons, 1948), pp. 7-8.

11. Jones, p. 8.

12. R. Buckminster Fuller, **Synergetics**; (New York: MacMillan Publishing Co., 1975), p. xxviii.

13. This becomes easier when it is realized that many popularly held ideas about the nature of life have been experimentally invalidated in recent years, as explained by Fuller, <u>op cit</u> p. xxx: "The supposed location of the threshold between animate and inanimate was methodically narrowed down by experimental science until it was confined specifically within the domain of virology. Virologists have ... found that no physical threshold does, in fact, exist between animate and inanimate ... Belated news of the elimination of this threshold must be interpreted to mean that whatever life must be, it has not been isolated and, thereby, identified as residual in the biological cell, as had been supposed by the false assumption that there was a separate physical phenomenon called animate within which life existed. The threshold between animate and inanimate has vanished."

14. See Chapter Two, Spirit or Self, as beyond mind, was included in the ancient texts. But the Buddhist source on which the present work is based does not consider this idea valid or necessary in its definition of life.

15. Rudolph Ballentine, **Diet and Nutrition** (Honesdale, PA: Himalayan International Institute, 1978), p. 579.

16. Most of the world's religions and modern science use similar triune principles to understand reality. See David Bohm in the **Enfolding-Unfolding Universe in the Holographic Paradigm and other Paradoxes**. Edited by Ken Wilber (Boulder, CO: Shambhala, 1982) pp 99-100.

17. For a discussion of the reasoning behind this view, see Marc Edmund Jones, <u>op cit</u>, pp. 211-234.

Bibliography

Airola, Paavo. **How To Get Well.** Phoenix: Health Plus Publishers, 1974.

Bailey, Liberty Hyde. **Hortus Third.** New York: MacMillan Publishing Co., 1976.

Bajracharya, Vaidya Mana Bajra. "Animals and Birds for Treatment" (unpublished paper).

Arthritis. Pamphlet. Kathmandu: Piyusavarsi Ausadhalaya Publisher, 1979.

"Ayurvedic Anatomy and Physiology" (unpublished paper).

"Ayurvedic Hygiene" (unpublished paper).

Ayurvedic Medicinal Plants and General Treatment. Kathmandu: Piyusavarsi Ausadhalaya Publishers, 1979.

"Ayurvedic Pharmacology" (unpublished paper).

"Ayurvedic Psychology" (unpublished paper).

"The Ayurvedic Science of Disease" (unpublished paper).

"The Ayurvedic Theory of Treatment" (unpublished paper).

"Breast Cancer" Kathmandu: Piyusavarsi Ausadhalaya Publishers, 1979.

The Eastern Theory of Diet. Edited by Alan K. Tillotson, Kathmandu: Piyusavarsi Ausadhalaya Publishers, 1978.

"First Anemia, Then Hepatitis" Pamphlet. Kathmandu: Piyusavarsi Ausadhalaya Publishers, 1978.

"Germs and Parasites" (unpublished paper).

"Minerals for Treatment" (unpublished paper).

"An Outline of Historical Background of Ayurveda" (unpublished paper).

"The Traditional Way of Ayurvedic Study" (unpublished paper).

"Tridosha Siddhanta, The Three Principles" (unpublished paper).

Ballentine, Rudolph. **Diet and Nutrition.** Honesdale: Himalayan International Institute, 1978.

Ballentine, Rudolph, Alan Hymes, and Swami Rama. **Science of Breath.** Honesdale: Himalayan International Institute, 1979.

Bhattacharyya, A.K. **Tridosha and Homeopathy.** Calcutta: Firma K.L. Mukhopadhyay, 1975.

Bhishagratna, K.L. **Susruta Samhita.** 3 volumes. New Delhi: Chowkhambra Sanskrit Series Office, 1976

Christopher, John. **School of Natural Healing.** Provo, Utah: BiWorld Publishers, Inc.

Conze, Edward. **Buddhism: Its Essence and Development.** New York: MacMillan Co., 1962.

Conze, Edward, et. al, eds. **Buddhist Texts Through the Ages.** New York: Harper and Row, 1964.

A Course in Miracles. New York: Coleman Graphics, 1977.

Dash, Bhagwan, **Fundamentals of Ayurvedic Medicine.** Delhi: Bensal Publishing, 1978.

Dash, Bhagwan, and R.K. Sharma, **Charaka Samhita.** 4 volumes. New Delhi: Chowkhambra Sanskrit Series Office, 1976.

Davis, F.A. **Taber's Cyclopedic Medical Dictionary.** Philadelphia: F.A. Davis Co., 1977.

Dwarkanath, P. **Introduction to Kayachikitsa.** Bombay: G.R. Bhatkal Popular Book Depot, 1959.

Evans, Geoffrey. **Medical Treatment Principles and Their Application.** London: Butterwork and Co., Ltd., 1951.

Fuller, Buckminster. **Synergetics.** New York: MacMillan Co., 1975.

Grieve, M. **A Modern Herbal.** 2 volumes. New York: Dover Publications, 1971.

Heinerman, John. **Science of Herbal Medicine.** Orem: BiWorld Publishers, 1979.

Jones, Marc Edmund. **Occult Philosophy.** Baltimore, Md.: Schneidereith and Sons, 1948.

Kushi, Michio. **The Book of Macrobiotics.** Boston: East-West Publications, 1977.

176

The Macrobiotic Way of Natural Healing. Boston: East-West Publications, 1978.

Oriental Diagnosis. London: Sunwheel Publications, 1978.

Kutumbia, O. **Ancient Indian Medicine.** New Delhi: Orient Longmans. Ltd., 1962.

Lad, Vasant. **Ayurveda: The Science of Self-Healing.** Santa Fe: The Lotus Press, 1984.

Murti, G. Srinavasa. **The Science and Art of Indian Medicine.** Adyar: Theosophical Press, 1931.

Nath, Sen Gupta. **The Ayurvedic System of Medicine.** Calcutta: R. Chatergee Publishing, 1926.

Rinpoche, Rechung. **Tibetan Medicine.** Los Angeles: University of California Press, 1976.

Tierra, Michael. **The Way of Herbs.** Santa Cruz: Unity Press, 1980.

For an additional list of books, contact::

National Library of Medicine, 8600 Rockville Pike, Bethesda, Md., 20894, 301-496-6308

INDEX

Diagrams and Tabulations

Correspondences between the Three Principles and
   the Body, The   27
Effects of the Seasons on the Three Major Energy
   Systems, The   87
Effects of the Six Tastes on the Three Major Energy
   Systems, The   67
Effects of the Tastes on the Three Major Energy
   Systems, The   97
Examples of Proper Meal Schedules   89
Identifying Characteristics of the Three Natures   40
Major Energy Systems and the Six Tastes   80
Model for a Non-Vegetarian Meal   77
Model for a Vegetarian Meal   77
Regular Diet, The   79
Specific Actions   69

A

Adityanath, 6
Air, x
Arthritis, 108ff.
Ashtanga Hridaya, 6
Ayurveda, definition of, 1;
   history, 11ff.;
   methodology, 9ff.;
   origin of, 2;
   principles, 18;
   purpose, 14

Agnivesa, 3
Artharva veda, 1
Ashtanga Ayurveda, 3
Atreya Punarvasu, 4

Bhela Samhita, 3
Breast Feeding, 91

Chakrapani, 3
Charaka, 2
Circulation, 92

Debate, 9
Digestion, 68

Earth, x
Eyes, Ears., Nose,
  Mouth & Throat, 5

Fire, x

Glandular cancer, 106

Harappa, 2
Health, definition of, 27
Herpes, 113
Hygiene, 89

Internal Medicine, 3

Janaka, 3

B
Breast Cancer, 91, 104ff.

C
Charaka Samhita, 2
Children's diseases, 5
Cooling, 67

D
Diets, for imbalance, 80ff.
Dridhabala, 4

E
Etiology, 53, 57ff.

F
Foods, antagonistic 87

G

H
Harita Samhita, 3
Heating, 67
Home Study, 10

I

J

179

Kapha, 20ff.
Kayachikitsa Tantra, 3

K

Kasyapa, 5

L

Life, definition, 41

M

Madhava Nidama, 4
Medical Conference, 14ff.
Medicines, specific, 69ff.
Mental Illness, 47
Mind, faculties of, 42ff.;
    states of, 44ff.

Meals, 88f.
Medical Instruction, 81ff.
Menstruation, 92
Metabolic Nature, 36f.
Mohenjo-daro, 2
Muscular Cancer, 106

N

Nagarjuna, 6
Nerve nature, 34ff.

Nau, 5
Nutritive Nature, 37ff.

O

Over-balance, 54ff.

P

Physical properties, 66
Plants, 72
Prakruti, x
Psychology, 32

Pitta, 18
Postgraduate study, 10
Precursor Symptoms, 59
Purusha, ix

R

Rejuvenation, 6ff.

Rohini, 100ff.

S

Salya Tantra, 4
Sanskrit, 9
Scirrhus cancer, 104
Spiritual Healing, 7ff.
Sushruta, 1
Symptoms, 60ff.

Samanya, 53ff.
Sarngadhara, 4
Seasons, 85ff.
Surgery, 4ff.
Susruta Samhita, 5

T

Tastes, 64ff., 78ff.
Toxicology, 6
Treatment, general, 96ff.;
    specific, 98ff.

Testing, 61
Toxins, 59, 98

U

Ulcerous Cancer, 106

V

Vagbhata, 4
Vedas, 2
Vijayaraksita, 4

Vata, 18
Videha Tantra, 5

W

Water, x